T0076243

# VETERINARIAN WORKFORCE ROLE IN DEFENSE AGAINST ANIMAL DISEASE

# ANIMAL SCIENCE, ISSUES AND PROFESSIONS SERIES

**Animal Genetics**
*Leopold J. Rechi*
*(Editor)*
2009. ISBN: 978-1-60741-844-3

**Primatology: Theories, Methods and Research**
*Emil Potocki and Juliusz Krasiński*
*(Editors)*
2009. ISBN: 978-1-60741-852-8

**Dolphins: Anatomy, Behavior and Threats**
*Agustin G. Pearce and Lucía M. Correa*
*(Editors)*
2010. ISBN: 978-1-60876-849-3

**The Integument of Dolphins**
*Wilfried Meyer*
2010. ISBN: 978-1-61668-254-5

**The Integument of Dolphins**
*Wilfried Meyer*
2010. ISBN: 978-1-61668-604-8

**Cognitive Visual Memory in Cats**
*V. M. Okujava, and T. A. Natishvili*
2010. ISBN: 978-1-61668-293- 3

**Cognitive Visual Memory in Cats**
*V. M. Okujava, and T. A. Natishvili*
2010. ISBN: 978-1-61668-612-3
(Online Book)

**Mycotoxicoses in Animals**
**Economically Important**
*Edlayne Gonçalez, Joana D'arc Felicio*
*and Simone Aquino*
*(Editors)*
2010. ISBN: 978-1-61668-195-1

**Whales and Dolphins: Behavior,**
**Biology and Distribution**
*Craig A. Murray*
2010. ISBN: 978-1-61668-693-2

**Whales and Dolphins: Behavior,**
**Biology and Distribution**
*Craig A. Murray*
2010. ISBN: 978-1-61668-805-9 (Online Book)

**Veterinarian Workforce Role in Defense**
**Against Animal Disease**
*Justin C. Bennett*
*(Editor)*
2010. ISBN: 978-1-60741-656-2

ANIMAL SCIENCE, ISSUES AND PROFESSIONS SERIES

# VETERINARIAN WORKFORCE ROLE IN DEFENSE AGAINST ANIMAL DISEASE

## JUSTIN C. BENNETT
### EDITOR

Nova Science Publishers, Inc.

*New York*

For permission to use material from this book please contact us:
Telephone 631-231-7269; Fax 631-231-8175
Web Site: http://www.novapublishers.com

**NOTICE TO THE READER**

LIBRARY OF CONGRESS CATALOGING-IN-PUBLICATION DATA

Veterinarian workforce role in defense against animal disease / editor, Justin C. Bennett.
    p. ; cm.
 Includes bibliographical references and index.
 ISBN 978-1-60741-656-2 (softcover)
  1. Veterinarians--Supply and demand--United States. 2. Communicable diseases in animals--United States. I. Bennett, Justin C.
    [DNLM: 1. Veterinary Medicine--manpower. 2. Animal Diseases--prevention & control. 3. Disease Outbreaks--veterinary. 4. Physician's Role. 5. Veterinarians--supply & distribution. SF 760.S64 V586 2009]
    SF623.V48 2009
    636.089'440973--dc22

                                                                            2009034183

*Published by Nova Science Publishers, Inc.*  ✦ *New York*

# CONTENTS

# PREFACE

## *United States Government Accountability Office*

## WHY GAO DID THIS STUDY

Veterinarians are essential for controlling zoonotic diseases—which spread between animals and humans—such as avian influenza. Most federal veterinarians work in the Departments of Agriculture (USDA), Defense (DOD), and Health and Human Services (HHS). However, there is a growing national shortage of veterinarians. GAO determined the extent to which (1) the federal government has assessed the sufficiency of its veterinarian workforce for routine activities, (2) the federal government has identified the veterinarian workforce needed during a catastrophic event, and (3) federal and state agencies encountered veterinarian workforce challenges during four recent zoonotic outbreaks. GAO surveyed 24 federal entities about their veterinarian workforce; analyzed agency workforce, pandemic, and other plans; and interviewed federal and state officials that responded to four recent zoonotic outbreaks.

## WHAT GAO RECOMMENDS

GAO is making recommendations to help ensure sufficient veterinarian capacity to protect public and animal health. In commenting on a draft of this report USDA, DOD, OPM, DHS, and Interior generally agreed with our recommendations. HHS generally concurred with the report, but disagreed with a 2007 FDA Advisory Committee report GAO cited, which said that FDA's Center of Veterinary Medicine is in a state of crisis.

# WHAT GAO FOUND

The federal government lacks a comprehensive understanding of the sufficiency of its veterinarian workforce. More specifically, four of five component agencies GAO reviewed have assessed the sufficiency of their veterinarian workforce to perform routine activities and have identified current or future concerns. This includes USDA's Animal and Plant Health Inspection Services (APHIS), Food Safety and Inspection Service (FSIS), and Agricultural Research Service (ARS); and DOD's Army. Current and future shortages, as well as noncompetitive salaries, were among the concerns identified by these agencies. HHS's Food and Drug Administration (FDA) does not perform such assessments and did not identify any concerns. In addition, at the department level, USDA and HHS have not assessed their veterinarian workforces across their component agencies, but DOD has a process for doing so. Moreover, there is no governmentwide effort to search for shared solutions, even though 16 of the 24 federal entities that employ veterinarians raised concerns about the sufficiency of this workforce. Further exacerbating these concerns is the number of veterinarians eligible to retire in the near future. GAO's analysis revealed that 27 percent of the veterinarians at APHIS, FSIS, ARS, Army, and FDA will be eligible to retire within 3 years.

Efforts to identify the veterinarian workforce needed for a catastrophic event are insufficient.Specifically, agencies' plans lack important elements necessary for continuing essential veterinarian functions during a pandemic, such as identifying which functions must be performed on-site and how they will be carried out if absenteeism reaches 40 percent—the rate predicted at the height of the pandemic and used for planning purposes. In addition, one federal effort to prepare for the intentional introduction of a foreign animal disease is based on the unrealistic assumption that all affected animals will be slaughtered, as the United States has done for smaller outbreaks, making the resulting veterinarian workforce estimates irrelevant. A second effort lacks crucial data, including data on how the disease would spread in wildlife. If wildlife became infected, as they have in the past, response would be greatly complicated and could require more veterinarians and different expertise.

Officials from federal and state agencies involved in four recent zoonotic disease outbreaks commonly cited insufficient veterinarian capacity as a workforce challenge. However, 10 of the 17 agencies that GAO interviewed have not assessed their own veterinarian workforce's response to individual outbreaks and are thus missing opportunities to improve future responses. Moreover, none of the entities GAO reviewed has looked across outbreaks to identify common workforce challenges and possible solutions.

## ABBREVIATIONS

| | |
|---|---|
| APHIS | Animal and Plant Health Inspection Service |
| ARS | Agricultural Research Service |
| CDC | Centers for Disease Control and Prevention |
| CSREES | Cooperative State Research, Education, and Extension Service |
| CVM | Center for Veterinary Medicine |
| DHS | Department of Homeland Security |
| DOD | Department of Defense |
| FDA | Food and Drug Administration |
| FEMA | Federal Emergency Management Agency |
| FSIS | Food Safety and Inspection Service |
| HHS | Department of Health and Human Services |
| HSPD | Homeland Security Presidential Directive |
| Interior | Department of the Interior |
| NADC | National Animal Disease Center |
| NAFV | National Association of Federal Veterinarians |
| NIH | National Institutes of Health |
| OIG | Office of Inspector General |
| OPM | Office of Personnel Management |
| SES | Senior Executive Service |
| USDA | Department of Agriculture |
| USGS | U.S. Geological Survey |

February 4, 2009 February 4, 2009
The Honorable Daniel K. Akaka

Chairman
Subcommittee on Oversight of Government Management, the Federal
Workforce, and the District of Columbia
Committee on Homeland Security and Governmental Affairs

Dear Mr. Chairman

Veterinarians play a vital role in the defense against animal diseases—
whether naturally or intentionally introduced—and these diseases can cause
serious harm to human health and the economy. For example, veterinarians
were at the forefront of the response to the 2001 United Kingdom outbreak of
foot-and-mouth disease, which resulted in the slaughter of more than 4 million
animals to control the outbreak, losses of over $5 billion to the food and
agriculture sectors, and comparable losses to the tourism industry.
Veterinarians are also essential for controlling zoonotic diseases, which are
diseases that spread between animals and humans. Zoonotic diseases are of
particular concern because, in recent years, about 75 percent of the newly
emerging infectious diseases affecting humans have originated in animals. For
example, over the past few years, a highly pathogenic strain of avian influenza
has killed millions of wild and domestic birds worldwide and infected over
400 people, more than half of whom have died. Health experts are concerned
that this virus could cause a pandemic if it develops the ability to spread
efficiently from human to human. Veterinarians also help prevent foodborne
illness, which humans can acquire, for example, from meat contaminated with
viruses or bacteria. Each year, about 76 million Americans contract foodborne
illnesses, and about 5,000 die.

However, there is a growing shortage of veterinarians nationwide,
particularly of veterinarians who care for animals raised for food, serve in
rural communities, and have training in public health, according to several
professional associations. This shortage has, according to the American
Veterinary Medical Association, placed the nation's food supply at risk and
could hinder efforts to protect humans from zoonotic diseases. The
veterinarian shortage is expected to worsen, partly as a result of space
constraints at the country's 28 veterinary colleges, which can graduate only
about 2,500 students a year combined, according to the American Association
of Veterinary Medical Colleges. The demand for veterinarians is expected to

increase, however. For example, the Bureau of Labor Statistics predicts that demand will increase by 35 percent from 2006 to 2016—from 62,000 full-time jobs to 84,000. Subsequently, the Congress enacted two pieces of legislation that address these concerns. In 2003, it enacted the National Veterinary Medical Services Act directing the Secretary of Agriculture to carry out a program to help repay school loans for veterinarians who agree to work in areas of need. In August 2008, the Congress passed the Higher Education Opportunity Act, which has provisions intended to increase the number of veterinarians in the workforce.

The federal government employs more than 3,000 veterinarians. Although this number represents a small portion of the federal workforce, these veterinarians play a crucial role in helping to protect people and the economy from animal diseases. More than 2,900 federal veterinarians work for component agencies within the Departments of Agriculture (USDA), Defense (DOD), and Health and Human Services (HHS). The 1,771 veterinarians at USDA have numerous functions, including the following:

- Animal and Plant Health Inspection Service (APHIS) veterinarians help protect and maintain the health of American livestock and poultry during production, and monitor wildlife populations for critical endemic and foreign animal diseases;
- Food Safety and Inspection Service (FSIS) veterinarians inspect animals at slaughter plants to help ensure the safety of meat and poultry products, and they also oversee the humane treatment of livestock during slaughter; and
- Agricultural Research Service (ARS) veterinarians research critical endemic and foreign animal diseases.

  DOD employs 841 veterinarians, the majority of whom work for the Army as active duty veterinarians or as part of the Army's veterinary reserve corps. These veterinarians are responsible for caring for service and research animals, ensuring food safety at military installations, and conducting intelligence work related to bioterrorism, among other things.

  HHS employs 316 veterinarians, whose functions include the following:

- Food and Drug Administration (FDA) veterinarians are responsible for ensuring that animal drugs are safe and effective, that animal feed is safe, and that food from medically treated animals is safe to eat.

They also help ensure the safety of food, drugs, and cosmetics, among other things;

- Centers for Disease Control and Prevention (CDC) veterinarians help promote human health by conducting research and investigating human disease outbreaks of animal origin. They also oversee the welfare of animals used in such research, as required by federal regulation.

Veterinarians work in other departments, such as the Department of the Interior (Interior), whose 24 veterinarians play a role in researching, diagnosing, and responding to wildlife diseases. The Department of Homeland Security (DHS) also employs veterinarians to, among other things, help develop national policy for defending the nation's agriculture and food supply against terrorist attacks and other emergencies. See appendix I for a list of veterinarian roles and responsibilities within the federal government.

As this list of responsibilities indicates, the federal veterinarian workforce plays a critical role in ensuring the safety of the U.S. food supply. However, we testified in 2008 that the staffing levels at FSIS—where veterinarians play an important role in helping to ensure the safety of our food supply and the humane treatment of animals during slaughter—have declined since 1995 despite an increasing budget, and some districts have experienced high vacancy rates among inspectors. This could impair enforcement of the Humane Methods of Slaughter Act of 1978 and of food safety regulations generally.[1] In addition, we have designated the federal oversight of food safety as a high-risk area of government operations because the current system is fragmented, causing inconsistent oversight, ineffective coordination, and inefficient use of resources.[2]

As with all professions in the federal government, departments and their component agencies are responsible for hiring and maintaining a veterinarian workforce sufficient to meet their missions. High-performing public organizations have found that maintaining a quality workforce requires them to systematically assess current and future workforce needs and formulate a long-term strategy to attract, retain, develop, and motivate employees.[3] The Office of Personnel Management (OPM) provides guidance and leadership intended to help build a high-quality and diverse federal workforce. Our prior work has identified the need for OPM to use its leadership position to help departments and agencies recruit and retain a capable and committed workforce.[4]

In this context, you asked us to determine the extent to which (1) the federal government has assessed the sufficiency of its veterinarian workforce for routine program activities, (2) the federal government has identified the veterinarian workforce needed during a catastrophic event, and (3) federal and state agencies encountered veterinarian workforce challenges during four recent zoonotic outbreaks.

To address the first objective, we identified and surveyed departments, component agencies, and other federal entities employing veterinarians to determine, among other things, the number, salaries, and roles and responsibilities of veterinarians, as well as the sufficiency of this workforce. We then selected component agencies within three departments for further analysis to determine the extent to which they assessed the sufficiency of their veterinarian workforce. We selected USDA, DOD, and HHS because these departments employ about 96 percent of federal veterinarians. Within these departments, we focused our veterinarian workforce assessment review on APHIS, FSIS, Army, and FDA, because these component agencies employ the most veterinarians. We also selected ARS for further review because it is USDA's chief scientific research agency and conducts research to solve agricultural problems of high national priority. We interviewed officials involved in workforce planning, as well as those that carry out program activities such as veterinarians working in slaughter plants. To address the second objective, we analyzed agency plans for continuing essential functions during a pandemic, and compared them with DHS national planning guidance, which identifies essential elements that federal departments and agencies should consider. We also reviewed veterinarian workforce outcomes from DHS's nationwide effort to assess the nation's preparedness for multiple, intentional introductions of foot-and-mouth disease. We selected a pandemic and intentional foot-and-mouth disease outbreak because these are two potential catastrophic events the White House Homeland Security Council has deemed critical for planning purposes. To address the third objective, we conducted semistructured interviews with selected officials from 17 federal and state agencies involved in responding to the following four recent zoonotic outbreaks:

- bovine tuberculosis in Michigan: a bacterial disease that spreads from deer to cattle;
- exotic Newcastle disease in California: a highly infectious virus that spread rapidly throughout poultry;

- monkeypox in Wisconsin: a virus not seen in the United States until 2003, when there was an outbreak in exotic pets and humans; and
- West Nile virus in Colorado: a disease that spread rapidly across the United States, infecting numerous species.

We focused our review on these outbreaks because they were most frequently recommended by federal officials as examples of zoonotic diseases, are still occurring or occurred since 2001, and affected various types of animals, among other things. Additional details about our scope and methodology are presented in appendix II.

We conducted this performance audit from September 2007 to February 2009, in accordance with generally accepted government auditing standards. Those standards require that we plan and perform the audit to obtain sufficient, appropriate evidence to provide a reasonable basis for our findings and conclusions based on our audit objectives. We believe that the evidence obtained provides a reasonable basis for our findings and conclusions based on our audit objectives.

## End Notes

[1] GAO, *Humane Methods of Handling and Slaughter: Public Reporting on Violations Can Identify Enforcement Challenges and Enhance Transparency*, GAO-08-686T (Washington, D.C.: April 17, 2008).

[2] GAO, *High-Risk Series: An Update*, GAO-09-271 (Washington, D.C.: January 2009).

[3] GAO, *Human Capital: Key Principles for Effective Strategic Workforce Planning*, GAO-04-39 (Washington, D.C.: Dec. 11, 2003).

[4] GAO, *Human Capital: Transforming Federal Recruiting and Hiring Efforts*, GAO-08-762T (Washington, D.C.: May 8, 2008).

In: Veterinarian Workforce Role in Defense...     ISBN: 978-1-60741-656-2
Editor: Justin C. Bennett                © 2010 Nova Science Publishers, Inc.

*Chapter 1*

# RESULTS IN BRIEF

## *United States Government Accountability Office*

Despite a growing shortage of veterinarians, the federal government does not have a comprehensive understanding of the sufficiency of its veterinarian workforce for routine program activities. Specifically, although four of five component agencies we reviewed have assessed their veterinarian workforces, little has been done to gain a broader, departmentwide perspective, and no assessment has been conducted governmentwide.

- At the component agency level, APHIS, FSIS, ARS, and Army assessments have each identified actual or potential veterinarian shortages. First, APHIS reported it has filled all of its veterinary positions but has identified a potential future shortage of, for example, veterinary pathologists, who diagnose animal diseases. In addition, 30 percent of APHIS' veterinarians will be eligible to retire by the end of fiscal year 2011. Second, FSIS has not been fully staffed over the past decade, according to agency officials. In fiscal year 2008, it had a goal of employing 1,134 veterinarians to carry out its mission of ensuring the safety of meat and poultry products, but it had 968 as of the end of that fiscal year—a 15 percent shortage. FSIS veterinarians working in slaughter plants told us that a lack of veterinarians has impaired the agency's ability to meet its food safety responsibilities, but FSIS headquarters officials told us this was not the case. In 2004, we recommended that FSIS periodically assess whether the level of resources dedicated to humane handling and slaughter activities is sufficient, but the agency has yet to demonstrate that they have done so. Third, ARS reported a 12 percent shortage of veterinarians. Officials told us the agency needed 65 veterinarians—most of them with a Ph.D.—to conduct critical animal disease research, such as detecting avian influenza and developing vaccines against it. However, in fiscal year 2008, ARS had only 57. Fourth, while the Army has filled all of its active-duty veterinarian positions, officials reported that the veterinary reserve corps is 12 percent short of its goal and identified an increasing demand for veterinary pathologists and medical intelligence specialists. In contrast to these four agencies, FDA does not regularly assess the sufficiency of its veterinarian workforce. FDA officials told us the agency has enough veterinarians to meet its responsibilities, despite a 2007 internal review that found its scientific workforce, including veterinarians, is inadequate and that FDA's Center for Veterinary Medicine is in a state of crisis.

- At the department level, neither USDA nor HHS has assessed its veterinarian workforce to gain a departmentwide perspective on trends and shared issues, whereas DOD has a process for doing so. USDA does not perform such assessments because, according to department-level officials, workforce planning is the responsibility of the component agencies. As a result, USDA's agencies compete against one another for a limited number of veterinarians. According to FSIS officials, APHIS is attracting veterinarians away from FSIS because the work at APHIS is more appealing, there are more opportunities for advancement, and the salaries are higher. HHS officials told us they do not assess veterinarian workforce needs departmentwide because veterinarians are not deemed mission critical for the department, even though they are critical to the missions of its component agencies that employ veterinarians.

- Governmentwide, no integrated approach exists for assessing the current and future sufficiency of the veterinarian workforce. Yet officials from 16 of the 24 component agencies and other federal entities that employ veterinarians told us they are concerned about the sufficiency of their veterinarian workforce. This includes four of the five key agencies where we focused our agency-level review. Further exacerbating these concerns is the number of veterinarians eligible to retire in the near future. Our analysis revealed that 27 percent of the veterinarians at APHIS, FSIS, ARS, Army, and FDA will be eligible to retire within 3 years. OPM officials told us they will initiate a governmentwide effort to address this issue if the departments demonstrate that a shortage exists. This could include allowing departments to expedite the hiring of veterinarians, as OPM has done in the past in the case of doctors and nurses.

We are making several recommendations to improve the federal government's ability to meet its routine veterinary responsibilities.

The federal government has undertaken efforts to identify the veterinarian workforce needed during two catastrophic events—a pandemic and multiple intentional introductions of foot-and-mouth disease. However, these efforts are insufficient because they are either incomplete, based on an infeasible planning assumption, or lacking in adequate data.

- Four of the five agencies we reviewed—APHIS, FSIS, ARS, and FDA—have developed pandemic plans that identify how they will continue essential functions, including those that veterinarians perform, during a pandemic that severely reduces the workforce. However, each plan lacks elements that DHS has deemed necessary. For example, FDA's plan does not identify which functions its veterinarians must perform on site, which can be performed remotely, or how the agency will conduct essential functions if a pandemic renders its leadership and essential staff unavailable. FDA officials told us they are updating their plan and will consider such gaps. The Army is still in the process of getting its pandemic plan approved and, therefore, we have not evaluated it.

- DHS has two efforts under way that involve identifying the workforce needed during a catastrophic outbreak of foot-and-mouth disease, which would require veterinarians to quickly diagnose and control the fast-moving disease in a large number of animals. The first effort is hindered by an infeasible planning assumption. Specifically, DHS is coordinating a long-term national effort that is based on the assumption, set forth by a White House Homeland Security Council working group, that the United States would slaughter all potentially exposed animals, as it has during smaller outbreaks of foreign animal diseases. However, DHS and USDA officials consider this approach infeasible for such a large outbreak and told us that although the planning effort is a valuable exercise for understanding the enormity of the resources needed to respond to such an event, any workforce estimates produced from this effort are not relevant.

The second effort is hindered by a lack of information. Specifically, DHS is modeling various foot-and-mouth disease outbreak scenarios in order to estimate the number and type of personnel needed for responding to foot-and-mouth disease by using vaccines, among other things. Vaccinating animals instead of slaughtering them to control the outbreak is a new strategy, which DHS and USDA officials believe may play an important role in controlling a catastrophic outbreak. However, the details of how this vaccine-based strategy would be implemented are not yet formalized, reducing the likelihood that workforce estimates will be accurate. In addition, the models do not yet factor in the potential for the disease to spread between livestock and wildlife. If wildlife became infected, as they have in some past outbreaks, control and eradication strategies would be greatly complicated and could require more veterinarians and different expertise. Agency officials recognize the importance of including wildlife for controlling and eradicating foot-and-mouth disease but told us that the data on how wildlife and livestock interact are limited.

We are making recommendations to improve the federal government's ability to identify the veterinarian workforce needed during a pandemic and to respond to a large-scale outbreak of foot-and-mouth disease.

The veterinarian workforce challenge most commonly cited by federal and state agencies involved in the four recent zoonotic outbreaks we reviewed was insufficient veterinarian capacity. Specifically, officials we interviewed at 12 of the 17 agencies involved in the recent outbreaks told us they did not have enough veterinarians to address these outbreaks while continuing to carry out their routine activities. Officials at numerous state agencies attribute this insufficient capacity to difficulty recruiting and retaining veterinarians because, among other things, the salaries they are able to offer are lower than those offered in the federal or private sectors. In addition, to control a demanding outbreak of exotic Newcastle disease in poultry in California in 2003, APHIS had to borrow more than 1,000 veterinarians from federal and state agencies around the country, as well as the private sector. This reduced the number of veterinarians available to respond to outbreaks of bovine tuberculosis in Michigan, monkeypox in Wisconsin, and West Nile virus in Colorado. Despite reports of insufficient veterinarian capacity during the four outbreaks, the agencies have not taken full advantage of two key opportunities to learn from past experience. First, 10 of the 17 agencies have not assessed their own veterinarian workforce's response to individual outbreaks, which our prior work has identified as a useful tool for improving response.[1] Second, none of the agencies have looked across outbreaks to identify common challenges. Consequently, the agencies are missing the opportunity to identify workforce challenges that have arisen during outbreaks and ways to address them in the future. Federal and state agency officials we spoke with generally agreed that it would be beneficial to conduct postoutbreak assessments. However, some agency officials told us that they are already having difficulty meeting their responsibilities and have not had time to do so. We are making recommendations to improve the ability of the federal government to help ensure the efficient and effective use of the veterinarian workforce during future zoonotic disease outbreaks.

In commenting on a draft of this report, USDA, DOD, OPM, DHS, and Interior generally concurred with the report's recommendations. However, DHS did not agree that veterinarian workforce estimates produced from one of its planning efforts are not relevant. HHS generally concurred with our report but disagreed with a 2007 FDA Advisory Committee report GAO cited, which said that FDA's Center of Veterinary Medicine is in a state of crisis. USDA, DOD, HHS, OPM, DHS, and Interior also provided additional information, comments, and clarifications on the report's findings that we have addressed, as appropriate, throughout the report.

## End Notes

[1] GAO, *Emergency Preparedness and Response: Some Issues and Challenges Associated with Major Emergency Incidents,* GAO-06-467T (Washington, D.C.: Feb. 23, 2006).

In: Veterinarian Workforce Role in Defense...     ISBN: 978-1-60741-656-2
Editor: Justin C. Bennett     © 2010 Nova Science Publishers, Inc.

*Chapter 2*

# BACKGROUND

## *United States Government Accountability Office*

High-performing public organizations have found that maintaining a quality workforce requires them to systematically assess current and future workforce needs and formulate a long-term strategy to attract, retain, develop, and motivate employees. While simple in theory, strategic planning can be difficult to carry out. Managers must, for example, acquire accurate information on the workforce, set goals for employee performance, and develop ways to measure that performance. According to our previous work, strategic workforce planning should involve certain key principles. Among these principles is the need to involve top management, employees, and other stakeholders in developing, communicating, and implementing a strategic workforce plan. Other principles include determining the critical skills that will be needed, developing strategies to address any gaps in these skills, building the capability needed to address educational and other requirements important to support workforce planning strategies, and monitoring and evaluating progress toward workforce goals.[1] However, federal agencies have for years lacked a strategic approach to workforce management. Consequently, since 2001, we have identified human capital management as a high-risk area needing urgent attention and transformation.[2]

OPM provides information and guidance on a wide range of strategies that departments and agencies can use to help strategically plan for and maintain a workforce sufficient to accomplish their missions. This includes standard retention and recruitment payments, such as recruitment incentives and student loan repayments. OPM can also authorize departments to use additional strategies to address workforce shortage situations should standard strategies prove insufficient. For example, OPM can approve higher salaries for individual positions in an occupation if the agency has difficulty staffing a position requiring an extremely high level of expertise that is critical to the agency's successful accomplishment of an important mission.

In addition to maintaining a workforce sufficient for routine functions, departments and agencies are directed by the President to ensure they can carry out essential functions during a "catastrophic event." Such a catastrophic event is any natural or man-made incident, including terrorism, that results in extraordinary levels of mass casualties, damage, or disruption severely affecting the population, infrastructure, environment, economy, national morale, and/or government functions. To do so, agencies must develop continuity of operation plans for emergencies that disrupt normal operations. Continuity planning includes identifying and establishing procedures to ensure vital resources are safeguarded, available, and accessible to support continuity operations. Vital resources are personnel, equipment, systems, infrastructures, supplies, and other assets required to perform an agency's essential functions. DHS's Federal Emergency Management Agency (FEMA) provides direction to the federal executive branch for developing continuity plans and programs, including pandemic plans.

For one type of catastrophic event, a pandemic that severely reduces the workforce, DHS has developed guidance that identifies specific elements agencies should consider as they plan to maintain essential services and functions. FEMA concluded that planning for a pandemic requires a state of preparedness that goes beyond normal continuity of operations planning. On March 1, 2006, FEMA first issued guidance to assist departments and agencies in identifying special considerations for protecting the health and safety of employees and maintaining essential functions and services during a pandemic. The *Implementation Plan for the National Strategy for Pandemic Influenza* recommends that organizations plan for a 40 percent absenteeism rate at the height of a pandemic. In addition, it called for department and agency pandemic plans to be completed by March 31, 2006.

Departments and agencies must also plan for other events that could place extraordinary demands on their workforce, such as a catastrophic outbreak of a foreign animal disease. In December 2003, the President issued a Homeland Security Presidential Directive (HSPD-8) to establish national policy to strengthen the preparedness of the United States to prevent and respond to terrorist attacks, major disasters, and other emergencies. As part of its efforts to meet HSPD-8, a White House Homeland Security Council working group developed National Planning Scenarios for 15 major events, including a biological attack with a foreign animal disease, foot-and-mouth disease. According to the scenario, terrorists introduce the disease in several locations and states simultaneously. The transportation of livestock spreads the contagious virus to surrounding states and, within 10 days of the attack, more than half of the states may be affected. Ultimately, almost half the nation's beef, dairy, and swine would be affected. These scenarios serve as the basis for assessing the nation's preparedness for such an event by defining tasks that may be required and the capabilities needed governmentwide to perform these tasks. Although not a prescription for the resources needed to achieve these capabilities, they are intended to help identify such resource needs and guide planning efforts. No single jurisdiction or agency will be expected to perform every task, so the response to a catastrophic event will require coordination among all levels of government. State and local agencies are typically the first to respond, but federal agencies become involved if state resources are overwhelmed. In certain catastrophic events, it becomes the responsibility of DHS to coordinate the federal response.

## End Notes

[1] See GAO-04-39 ; GAO, *Human Capital: Insights for U.S. Agencies from Other Countries' Succession Planning and Management Initiatives*, GAO-03-914 (Washington, D.C.: Sept. 15, 2003).

[2] See *GAO-09-271* .

In: Veterinarian Workforce Role in Defense...      ISBN: 978-1-60741-656-2
Editor: Justin C. Bennett                © 2010 Nova Science Publishers, Inc.

*Chapter 3*

# THE FEDERAL GOVERNMENT LACKS A COMPREHENSIVE UNDERSTANDING OF THE SUFFICIENCY OF ITS VETERINARIAN WORKFORCE

## *United States Government Accountability Office*

Four of the five key agencies that employ veterinarians—APHIS, FSIS, ARS, and Army—regularly assess the sufficiency of their veterinarian workforces for routine program activities, and all four identified existing or potential shortages. FDA does not perform such assessments. At the department level, USDA and HHS have not assessed their veterinarian workforces across their component agencies, whereas DOD has delegated this task to the Army. Finally, there is no governmentwide assessment of the veterinarian workforce. Specifically, OPM has not conducted a governmentwide effort to address current and future veterinarian shortages identified by component agencies, and efforts by the Congress to address the national shortage have thus far had minimal impact.

# FOUR OF FIVE AGENCIES HAVE IDENTIFIED EXISTING AND POTENTIAL VETERINARIAN SHORTAGES

APHIS, FSIS, ARS, and Army conduct regular workforce assessments. While APHIS reported it does not currently have a shortage, it identified a potential future shortage. FSIS, ARS, and Army have identified both existing and potential future shortages. FDA does not conduct such assessments, but officials there told us the veterinarian workforce is adequate to meet its responsibilities. Our work has shown that agencies should be held accountable for the ongoing monitoring and refinement of human capital approaches to recruit and hire a capable and committed federal workforce.

## APHIS

APHIS reported that none of its six units that employ veterinarians has identified a current shortage, but officials told us they are concerned about the future size and skills of the veterinarian workforce. First, the agency reported that 30 percent of its veterinarians will be eligible to retire by the end of fiscal year 2011, potentially creating a serious shortage. This is consistent with our previous work where we reported that one-third of federal career employees on board at the end of fiscal year 2007 are eligible to retire between spring 2008 and 2012.[1] In addition, APHIS is concerned that it will be unable to maintain an adequate workforce of veterinary pathologists. This is consistent with a report by the United States Animal Health Association, which found a shortage of over 40 percent nationwide. An APHIS laboratory director told us that veterinary pathologists are integral to work conducted in APHIS diagnostic laboratories, including work on diseases that threaten animal and human health. For example, APHIS veterinary pathologists work on bovine spongiform encephalopathy, a fatal degenerative disease—commonly known as mad cow disease—that has been linked to at least 165 human deaths worldwide. APHIS also identified a need to maintain a veterinarian workforce with sufficient expertise to help protect livestock and the nation's food supply from foreign animal diseases. We reported in 2005 that many U.S. veterinarians lack the training needed to identify such diseases, whether naturally or intentionally introduced.[2] Finally, after the terrorist attacks of 2001, USDA's responsibilities were broadened to enhance the ability of the United States to manage domestic incidents. As such, in addition to being the lead for coordinating any response efforts to incidents involving an animal disease, APHIS will now also play a supporting role in incidents not directly related to animal diseases. For example, APHIS veterinarians may be called upon to assist in ensuring the safety and security of the commercial food supply or for caring for livestock stranded in hurricanes and floods. These increased responsibilities raise concerns about the ability of veterinarians to respond to multiple, simultaneous events, according to agency officials.

APHIS has supported training opportunities to help overcome some of these projected skill gaps. The agency has also set a goal of recruiting at all veterinary colleges and working with universities to help them include relevant training in their course offerings. In addition, APHIS uses bonuses to attract and maintain its veterinarian workforce. During the first 9 months of fiscal year 2008, it provided one retention and one relocation bonus to veterinarians, totaling $41,654.

## FSIS

Over the past decade, FSIS has not had a sufficient number of veterinarians and remains unable to overcome this shortage, according to FSIS officials. The agency's goal was to have 1,134 veterinarians on staff in fiscal year 2008, but it fell short of that by 166 veterinarians, or 15 percent. Moreover, since fiscal year 2003, the FSIS veterinarian workforce has decreased by nearly 10 percent—from 1,073 to 968. The majority of these veterinarians work in slaughter plants. Federal law prohibits slaughtering livestock or poultry at a plant that prepares the livestock or poultry for human consumption for use in interstate commerce unless the animals have been examined by USDA inspectors and requires the humane slaughtering and handling of livestock at such plants. In implementing federal law, each slaughter plant is covered by one or more FSIS veterinarians to, among other things, ensure the safety and quality of meat and poultry products and the humane treatment of livestock during slaughter. Agency data from the past 5 years reveal that vacancy rates for veterinarian positions in slaughter plants vary by location and year, from no vacancy to as many as 35 percent of the positions vacant.

FSIS headquarters officials and veterinarians working in slaughter plants differed on the impact of this shortage. Headquarters officials told us that, despite the shortage, the agency has been able to meet its food safety and other responsibilities by redistributing the workforce. For example, in some cases, FSIS has assigned one veterinarian to several slaughter plants or assigned only one to plants that previously had two. In contrast, several veterinarians working in slaughter plants told us that, because of inadequate staffing, they are not always able to meet their responsibilities and perform high-quality work. For example, veterinarians told us they cannot always verify crucial sanitation and security checks of the plant or promptly log data on animal diseases and welfare.

In early 2008, veterinarians also told us they did not always have time to ensure the humane treatment of livestock. Inhumane treatment triggered an investigation that led to the largest beef recall in U.S. history. More specifically, in February 2008, the Humane Society of the United States released videos to the public that documented abuse of cattle awaiting slaughter at a plant in Chino, California. These alleged abuses, which took place in the fall of 2007, included electrically shocking nonambulatory "downer" cattle, spraying them with high-pressure water hoses, and ramming them with a forklift in an apparent attempt to force them to rise for slaughter. These acts are not only cruel, they pose a risk to the safety of the food supply, because downer animals are known to be at greater risk for bovine spongiform encephalopathy. FSIS regulations require that downer cattle be separated to await disposition by an inspector, even if they become nonambulatory after an inspector has approved the animal for slaughter during the preslaughter inspection. On February 1, 2008, the plant voluntarily ceased operations pending investigation by FSIS into the alleged abuses. On February 17, 2008, the plant announced that it was voluntarily recalling approximately 143 million pounds of raw and frozen beef products because of its failure to notify FSIS of the downer cows and the remote possibility that the beef being recalled could cause adverse health effects if consumed. The release of the videos by the Humane Society led congressional committees and USDA to question how such events could have occurred at a plant in which FSIS inspectors were assigned. At the request of the Secretary of Agriculture, USDA's Office of Inspector General (OIG) is leading a criminal investigation that is ongoing at the time of this report. In addition, OIG conducted an audit of FSIS's controls over preslaughter activities and reported in November 2008 that controls to demonstrate the sufficiency and competency of FSIS' personnel resources could be strengthened to minimize the chance that such events could recur, among other things.[3]

Veterinarians and other FSIS officials we interviewed told us that, at the time of the incident, only one veterinarian was assigned to the plant that was the source of the recall, whereas two had been assigned in past years. Two veterinarians were needed, according to these officials, because the plant processed "cull" dairy cows, which are no longer used for milk production. These cows are generally older and in poorer condition than other livestock and thus require more frequent veterinary inspection. In the wake of this incident, FSIS required veterinarians to spend more time verifying the humane treatment of animals. However, veterinarians told us that this exacerbated the difficulty of completing their other work. In 2004, we made recommendations aimed at ensuring that FSIS can make well-informed estimates about the inspection resources—including veterinarians—needed to enforce the Humane Methods of Slaughter Act of 1978.[4] Specifically, we recommended that FSIS periodically assess whether the level of resources dedicated to humane handling and slaughter activities is sufficient, but the agency has yet to demonstrate that they have done so.

FSIS officials told us that there are several reasons for the agency's ongoing shortage of veterinarians. For example, most veterinarians do not want to work in the unpleasant environment of a slaughterhouse. Furthermore, veterinarians are trained to heal animals, but FSIS veterinarians are hired to oversee the slaughter of animals. The job can also be physically and emotionally grueling, and many of the plants are in remote and sometimes undesirable locations. In addition, as a result of staff shortages, there is little opportunity to take time off for training that could lead to promotion. Finally, FSIS veterinarians told us that their salaries do not sufficiently compensate for the working conditions and are low relative to those of other veterinarians. According to OPM's Central Personnel Data File, the mean annual salary for FSIS veterinarians in 2007 was $77,678; in contrast, the mean salary for private-practice veterinarians was $115,447 in 2007, according to the most recent data from the American Veterinary Medical Association. In commenting on a draft of this report, FSIS officials added that there is a lack of public health and food-safety emphasis in veterinary schools.

FSIS has taken several steps to address the shortage. For example, it awarded 35 recruitment bonuses totaling more than $583,000 in the first 9 months of fiscal year 2008. FSIS also has internship programs that have, according to agency officials, increased awareness and generated interest in veterinarian work at the agency. For example, over the past 5 years, FSIS has established agreements with 16 veterinary schools to provide volunteer training opportunities to veterinary students with an interest in food safety and public health. In fiscal year 2008, there were 26 participants in the program, compared with only 1 when the program began in 2003. Two participants have thus far returned to FSIS for full-time employment after graduation. FSIS also has a paid veterinary student program that is designed to provide experience directly related to the student's educational program and career goals. Since 2002, when FSIS began tracking this program, 77 students have participated, and 6 have become full-time employees. In addition, FSIS has sought special hiring authorities from OPM. For example, in July 2008, the agency was delegated authority to hire a limited number of retirees at full salary instead of at the reduced salary required for those with annuity income. Officials told us they hope this will encourage retired veterinarians to join FSIS, but, as of the date of this report, no retirees have been hired through this program. FSIS intends to track the effectiveness of this special hiring authority. Moreover, FSIS has proposed implementing a demonstration project that would allow the agency to test a pay system that offers more competitive salaries to veterinarians, among others. OPM requires that agencies undertaking such a project provide OPM with an analysis of the impact of the project results in relation to its objectives. OPM officials told us the project may be implemented in July 2009. Finally, OPM has in the past granted FSIS the ability to make immediate job offers to veterinarians without following prescribed competitive procedures, which can slow the hiring process. This "direct-hire authority" expired in 2007 and was not renewed at that time because, according to FSIS officials, USDA did not provide the expiration notification to FSIS. We were recently informed that USDA received approval from OPM on November 25, 2008, for direct hire for FSIS veterinarians lasting through December 31, 2009. However, FSIS officials raised concerns about the length of time of the authority, among other things, stating that it takes 5 to 6 months to renew this authority.

## ARS

ARS employed 57 veterinarians in fiscal year 2008, 12 percent short of its goal of 65. It has reported similar shortages throughout the last 5 years. Although veterinarians represent a small share of the ARS workforce (about 1 percent of more than 4,300 scientists and research technicians), the agency considers them critical to its mission. According to ARS officials, a sufficient veterinarian workforce is important to the quality and breadth of research ARS is able to conduct. For example, ARS would not have been able to conduct its research on the detection of avian influenza and development of vaccines

As other possible pinning agencies, the jogs on the dislocation lines are considered. The jogs are short dislocation segments which make the main dislocation line in a zigzag form. The jog cannot easily be moved by external stress and can be a pinning agency [16]. The jogs are generated on the dislocation line by a thermal activation process, and thus the number of jogs increases and their separation distance decreases with increasing temperature, and vice versa. Thus, the behavior shown in figure 11 can be explained by the idea of jog pinning. Meanwhile, the amplitude dependent behavior is seen in a higher level of input sound $s$ (dB) as shown in figure 12. The abscissa is the relative value of the amplitude. The results are well explained by the hysteresis-type loss caused from the jog-pinning. Inserted figures show the frequency dependence of IF. All curves in the figures represent theoretical ones. More quantitative discussion can be seen in the original article [14].

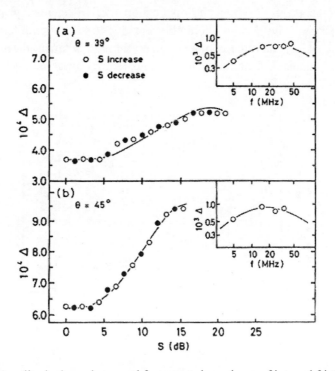

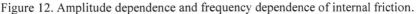

Figure 12. Amplitude dependence and frequency dependence of internal friction.

By observing the overdamped resonance curve, the dislocation density $\Lambda$ in the specimen can be determined. The temperature of a specimen $T_i$ is suddenly decreased and kept constant at $T_f$, and the change of $\Lambda$ with time $t$ is observed. The results of such an experiment are shown in figure 13. These results can be explained as follows. The dislocations are in an equilibrium configuration in a crystal at a certain temperature. Then, when the temperature is changed the dislocations move in order to take a new equilibrium configuration. It happens that the moving dislocations meat other ones and can be annihilated. Thus, $\Lambda$ decreases with time $t$, and the relation between the two can be

$$\Lambda \propto \exp(-Rt), \tag{21}$$

where $R$ is the reaction rate for the dislocation-dislocation annihilation process. The curves in figure 13 are the fitted ones, and the values of $R$ are determined. It is found that $R$ value is almost independent of the final or keeping temperature $T_f$. When the dislocation motion occurs by a thermal-activation process, the $R$ value should be sensitive to the keeping temperature. Thus, we consider that the motion occurs through a quantum-mechanical tunneling mechanism. Detailed analysis concerned is made along this line as shown in original article [15].

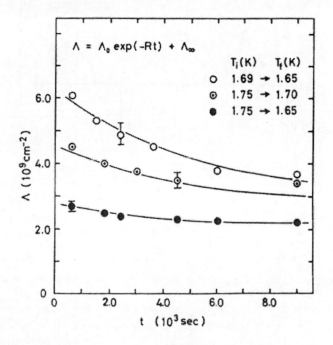

Figure 13. Change of dislocation density with time.

$$\Lambda = \Lambda_0 + K/[1 - (T/T_0)], \tag{22}$$

where $K$ and $T_0$ are constants. The determined values of $T_0$ and the melting temperature $T_M$ are as shown below:

20.5 cm$^3$/mole crystal: $T_0 = 1.78$ K, $T_M = 1.86$ K,
19.2 cm$^3$/mole crystal: $T_0 = 2.53$ K, $T_M = 2.52$ K. $\tag{23}$

It can be seen that the temperature $T_0$ is definitely lower than $T_M$ in the first kind crystal. It is remembered that the quantum-mechanical character can be more pronounced in the first kind crystal since its molar volume is larger.

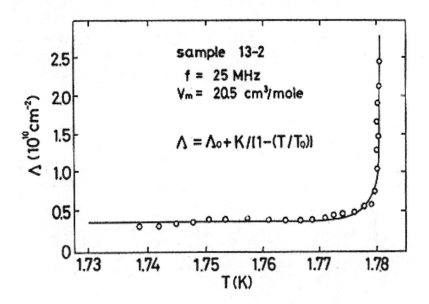

Figure 15. Temperature dependence of dislocation density in helium.

Here, we recall the dislocation theory of melting and liquid state [20]. The liquid is considered as a state containing a high density of dislocations. According to the idea of the theory, it is possible that dislocations are spontaneously produced when the temperature is raised to the temperature close to the melting point. The experimental data obtained presently suggest that the theory can be acceptable. However, we cannot present the meaning of Eq. (22) we obtained, which is at present merely an empirical expression.

# E. MELTING OF HELIUM CRYSTAL

Sound attenuation measurement has been carried out in helium crystals at temperatures below and above the melting temperature [17]. The specimens used are the same as those adopted in the previous study. The overall features of the melting and freezing of a crystal are shown in figure 14, where the solid curves are guide lines. The attenuation in the solid increases gradually and then rapidly with temperature below the melting point. After that the attenuation in the liquid decreases rapidly and then gradually. When the temperature of the liquid is lowered, similar attenuation changes occur. However, a large amount of supercooling can be seen as shown in the figure. The anomalous sound behavior such as a rapid change of sound velocity near the melting point is generally observed in usual materials [18, 19], and this phenomenon is not a special characteristic of helium crystal. The remarkable supercooling is also not special for helium crystal, since such a phenomenon is always observed in high purity materials. The large amount of supercooling seen in the helium crystal means that the crystal is very pure.

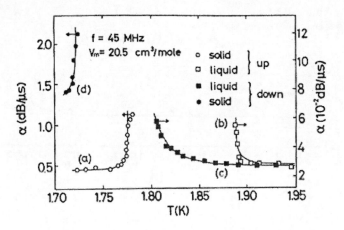

Figure 14. Temperature dependence of ultrasonic attenuation in melting and freezing .helium.

In the following, the premelting region of the solid is solely considered. As previously shown, the overdamped resonance can be seen in helium crystals in the frequency dependence of IF, and the dislocation density can be determined by analyzing the data. Figure 15 shows that the dislocation density $\Lambda$ increases gradually and then rapidly with temperature in the premelting region. The behavior is well represented by the formula against it, or on the transmission of bovine tuberculosis, without its veterinarians' skills and experience.

ARS officials told us it is difficult to attract and retain veterinarians because the agency requires its research veterinarians and senior program leaders who are veterinarians to have a Ph.D. in animal sciences or a related field, as well as a veterinary degree, and there is a limited pool of candidates for these positions. A recent report by the National Academy of Sciences identified a declining interest in veterinary research among veterinary students as a cause of a shortage of Ph.D. veterinarians. In addition, ARS officials told us the agency cannot compete with many of the salaries offered in the private sector. In 2007, the mean salary for ARS veterinarians was $102,081, according to OPM's Central Personnel Data File. This is about $28,000 less than the mean salary reported by the American Veterinary Medical Association for veterinarians with a Ph.D. working at universities and colleges and about $96,000 less than those working in industry with similar qualifications, such as at pharmaceutical companies.

To address its shortage of Ph.D. veterinarians, ARS provided six recruitment or retention bonuses to its veterinarians totaling $48,313 in the first 9 months of fiscal year 2008. The agency also created a tuition program in 2003, but participation has been limited. Only four individuals have been hired through the tuition program, and only two remained with the agency, according to officials. Under this program, ARS hires veterinarians without a Ph.D. and pays tuition and other educational costs while they earn this degree. Officials told us that the lack of success is most likely due to low salaries at ARS. In addition, the agency is reluctant to use this program because it diverts funding from the hiring of employees already qualified and ready to work.

## Army

The Army reported that it filled its 446 authorized active-duty veterinarian positions, but that its veterinary reserve corps is not at full strength. Specifically, the Army only filled 173 of its 197 reserve positions in fiscal year 2008, a 12 percent shortage. According to the Army's analysis, the reserve corps has been at less than full strength since fiscal year 2005. These veterinarians commit to part-time training and to being deployed to full-time active duty when needed. The shortage means there is not a sufficient pool of veterinarians that can be called into active duty as the need arises. This is a concern, according to the official responsible for assessing Army veterinarian workforce needs, because the Army's need for veterinarian services is increasing due to growing concerns over bioterrorism, intentional contamination of the food supply, emerging zoonotic diseases, and due to operational requirements, such as agricultural reconstruction in Afghanistan and Iraq, among other things. This official told us that recruitment into the reserves has been a problem because of the length, frequency, and uncertainty of deployments, which, in some cases has also resulted in veterinarians losing their jobs or suffering financial hardships. However, he told us that recent changes to the reserve corps program—such as decreasing the length of deployment from 1 year to 180 days, and making additional incentives available to veterinarians in the reserves—have helped strengthen the capacity of the veterinary reserve corps.

Officials also told us they are concerned about a growing need for certain special veterinary skills. For example, there is an increasing demand for Army veterinary pathologists, who are essential for interpreting test results from animals used in drug and vaccine research. The official responsible for assessing Army veterinarian workforce needs told us the Army has yet to formally assess this need. Other Army veterinarians conduct medical intelligence work for DOD's Defense Intelligence Agency, where officials told us they are concerned about the difficulty of recruiting veterinarians with appropriate skills to meet a growing need to, among other things, collect and analyze data on animal diseases that could be used in a terrorist attack. Veterinarians are important to such work because, according to these officials, the majority of diseases considered to be potential bioterrorism agents are animal diseases that could also affect humans. They told us that while the agency is working to expand its workforce capabilities to address bioterrorism, there is a concern that the growing demand for veterinarian capabilities may outpace the growth of the Army's workforce.

The primary reason for the Army's success in maintaining its active-duty veterinarian workforce is a scholarship program, according to the official responsible for assessing Army veterinarian workforce needs. This program targets veterinary students and pays their tuition and fees to veterinary school in exchange for a commitment to (1) serve as a veterinarian in the Army for 3 years and (2) serve an additional 5 years either in active duty or in the Army reserve program. In fiscal year 2008, the Army reported it had 106 qualified applicants for 47 scholarships. According to the official, the program is successful because it targets students before they accumulate school-related debt. Veterinary students graduate with more than $106,000 in debt, on average, according to the American Veterinary Medical Association. In addition, the funding for this program is directed specifically by congressional committees, separate from funds the Army uses to hire veterinarians.

## FDA

FDA officials reported that the agency has not assessed the sufficiency of its veterinarian workforce, but they told us that the workforce is sufficient to meet its responsibilities. However, a 2007 report by an FDA Advisory Committee found that FDA cannot fulfill its mission because of an insufficient scientific workforce.[5] More specifically, the report states that FDA's scientific workforce has remained static while its workload has increased, and that FDA's Center for Veterinary Medicine (CVM) is in a state of crisis. This center employs nearly two-thirds of FDA's 152 veterinarians and is responsible for ensuring the safety of veterinary drugs and regulating animal feed, among other things. An author of the report told us that veterinarians enter FDA employment lacking necessary skills and experience to examine the wide variety of veterinary products that require FDA approval and that FDA needs to better train its veterinarians to review the many diverse products under its jurisdiction. FDA officials told us the agency is currently undertaking significant reforms to address fundamental concerns in the report. For example, FDA reported it hired more than 1,000 scientists in order to build a more robust workforce, and it created the position of Chief Scientist to improve coordination of science planning and execution across the agency. However, FDA did not tell us how these reforms address the identified veterinarian skill gaps.

Although FDA officials said the veterinarian workforce is sufficient, CVM officials recently told us that as a result of new obligations, the center hired 26 veterinarians in 2008 to fill vacancies. This represents a 17 percent increase in FDA's overall veterinarian workforce in 2008, and it plans to hire more. The additional staff will enhance FDA's ability to review generic animal drug submissions, among other things, according to these officials. In addition, in commenting on a draft of this report, OPM informed us that it is currently reviewing a request for direct-hire authority from FDA to fill veterinary positions. According to OPM, this request is based on a severe shortage of candidates and it is projected that this authority may be granted through December 31, 2010. CVM also plans to develop an internship program for entry-level veterinarians and other scientists in order to develop a qualified talent pool from which to draw permanent employees. Further, these officials said that, as a result of recent participation in interagency efforts to protect the nation's food supply, CVM has begun to analyze the gap between its current resources and its needs.

# DEPARTMENTS HAVE DONE LITTLE TO ASSESS THE SUFFICIENCY OF THEIR VETERINARIAN WORKFORCES ACROSS THEIR COMPONENT AGENCIES

Even though their component agencies identified concerns about their veterinarian workforces, officials from both USDA and HHS told us that they have not undertaken a departmentwide assessment of these workforces to gain a broader perspective on trends and shared issues. In contrast, DOD has a process for such an assessment. Our prior work has found that top-level management needs to be involved in order for strategic workforce planning to be effective.[6]

## USDA

Although USDA regularly collects veterinarian workforce data from its component agencies that employ veterinarians, it does not use this information to assess the sufficiency of the veterinarian workforce departmentwide. Department officials told us that workforce assessment is the responsibility of the agencies. Because USDA delegates this responsibility, it appears to be unaware of the scope of the workforce problems facing its agencies. For example, in its fiscal year 2007 human capital management report, USDA reported that its agencies had met or surpassed certain veterinarian workforce goals but made no mention of the shortages that FSIS and ARS identified in their workforce reports. USDA officials agreed that the report did not capture this critical information and that future reports should address the shortages. One result of this lack of department-level involvement is that USDA agencies compete against one another for veterinarians instead of following a departmentwide strategy to balance the needs of the agencies. According to FSIS officials, APHIS is attracting veterinarians away from FSIS because the work at APHIS is more appealing, there are more opportunities for advancement, and the salaries are higher. Indeed, our analysis shows that veterinarians are more concentrated in lower grade levels at FSIS than at APHIS (see figure 1). Moreover, according to OPM's Central Personnel Data File, the mean annual salary for veterinarians at FSIS in 2007 was about $78,000, the lowest among the three key USDA agencies (see figure 2). According to an APHIS human resources official, the agency hired 75 veterinarians from FSIS between fiscal years 2003 and 2007, 17 percent of total new APHIS veterinarians hired.

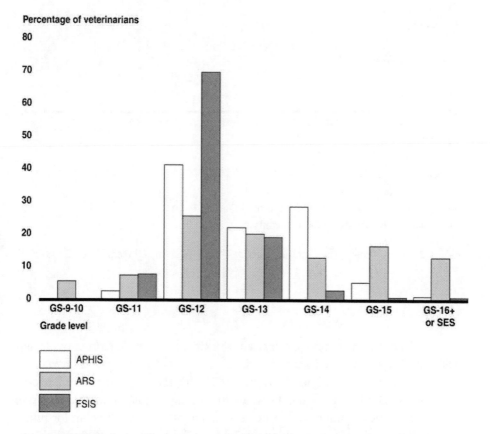

Source: GAO analysis of agency survey responses.
Note: Federal agency grade levels represent ascending rates of basic pay, from GS-1 through GS-15, above which is the Senior Executive Service (SES).

Figure 1. Percentage of Veterinarian Grade Levels by Key USDA Agencies in Fiscal Year 2008

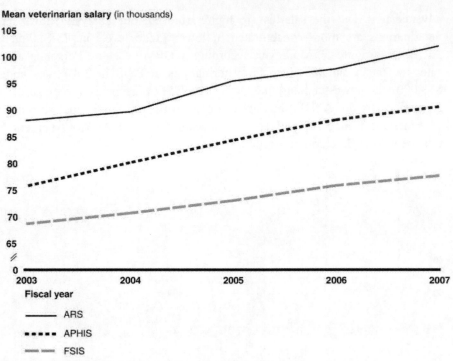

Source: GAO analysis of Central Personnel Data File data.
Note: Data in this figure contains locality pay.

Figure 2. Mean Veterinarian Salaries by Key USDA Agencies, Fiscal Years 2003-2007

## HHS

HHS neither assesses veterinarian workforce needs departmentwide nor has it instructed any of its component agencies that employ veterinarians—FDA, CDC, and the National Institutes of Health (NIH)—to assess their own workforces. HHS is thus not fully aware of the status of the veterinarian workforce at these component agencies and cannot strategically plan for future veterinarian needs. If it were able to provide such planning, it might be able to help FDA address workforce concerns raised in the 2007 *FDA Science and Mission at Risk* report. However, senior HHS strategic workforce planning officials we spoke with were unaware of the report.

HHS officials told us that departmental leadership in workforce planning is important. In fact, they said the department is in the preliminary stages of developing a strategic departmentwide approach to workforce planning for certain professions. This effort will initially focus on workforce assessments for specific occupations, such as nurses and medical doctors. HHS officials told us they will not initially include veterinarians in this effort, because veterinarians are not deemed mission critical for the department, even though they are critical to the missions of FDA, CDC, and NIH. However, HHS officials said that this effort does not preclude agencies from assessing their own veterinarian workforce needs and sharing that information with the department. HHS officials also told us that because the department is expected to provide veterinary medical care and support during public health and medical disasters that warrant a coordinated federal response, it is critical that appropriate veterinary resources are identified and maintained. Furthermore, these officials told us that efforts are under way at the component agency level to address the national veterinary shortage. Specifically, CDC, in collaboration with Emory University, has developed a residency program designed to provide comprehensive training in laboratory animal medicine to better prepare veterinarians for working in laboratory research facilities at CDC and across the nation. In addition, in 2006 and 2008 CDC sponsored a "Veterinary Student Day" to promote public health careers for veterinarians.

## DOD

Unlike USDA and HHS, DOD has a process for assessing veterinarian workforce needs departmentwide. It has given this responsibility to the Army, which employs 89 percent of DOD veterinarians, with the remaining veterinarians working as public health officials for the Air Force. The Army assesses not only the number and type of veterinarians it will need but also what will be needed for the other services. For example, Army veterinarians are routinely assigned to care for working dogs and other animals at Army, Navy, Air Force, and Marine bases. Army veterinarians also conduct medical intelligence activities at the Defense Intelligence Agency. As the executive agency charged with assessing veterinarian workforce requirements for DOD, the Army takes all of these needs into consideration, then forwards the assessment results to DOD, which integrates them with overall workforce planning.

# THERE IS NO GOVERNMENTWIDE ASSESSMENT OF THE VETERINARIAN WORKFORCE

No effort is being made to assess the sufficiency of the veterinarian workforce governmentwide. This is problematic because the majority (67 percent) of the 24 component agencies and other federal entities that employ veterinarians told us they have concerns about their veterinarian capabilities. OPM has not conducted a governmentwide effort to address current and future veterinarian shortages identified by component agencies, as it has done for other professions, and efforts by the Congress to address the national shortage have thus far had minimal impact.

Sixteen of the 24 component agencies and other entities employing veterinarians reported concerns about their veterinarian workforce (see table 1). For example, several agencies reported that they lack veterinarian expertise required to fully meet agency responsibilities, such as addressing wildlife disease outbreaks.

**Table 1. Agency Concerns about Sufficiency of the Federal Veterinarian Workforce**

| Department | Component agency/other federal entity | Examples of concerns reported by component agency/other federal entity |
|---|---|---|
| Department of Agriculture | Animal and Plant Health Inspection Service | Thirty percent of its veterinarians will be eligible to retire by the end of fiscal year 2011, and it may be diffi-cult to maintain enough veterinarians with expertise in pathology and fore-ign animal disease in the future. Res-ponsibilities have also increased in recent years, raising concerns that there will not be sufficient veteran-arian capacity if multiple emergen-cies occur at once. |
| | Food Safety and Inspection Service | Veterinarian workforce falls short of agency goal by 15 percent due, in part, to unpleasant environment, grueling work, and low salary. |
| | Agricultural Research Service | Veterinarian workforce falls short of agency goal by 12 percent. There is a limited number of qualified veterinarians and agency salaries are not competitive with private sector. |

Table 1. (Continued)

| Department | Component agency/other federal entity | Examples of concerns reported by component agency/other federal entity |
|---|---|---|
| | Cooperative State Research, Educ-ation, and Exten-sion Service | One of the four veterinarian positions is vacant, stressing the agency's ability to oversee funds for a national network of laboratories that diagnose and track animal diseases. |
| Department of Defense | Army | Veterinary reserve corps falls short by 12 percent. Also, the number of active-duty veterinarian positions has remained relatively static despite increasing demands across the Army's mission, including in medical |
| | | intelligence, food safety and defense, agricultural reconstruction efforts in Iraq and Afghanistan, and emerging zoonotic diseases. |
| | Air Force | Not enough veterinarians choose to join the Air Force because of the service commitment, and the salary is not competitive. Air Force officials are concerned they might not be able to fully meet the agency's public health mission, which includes ensuring food safety and tracking infectious diseases on Air Force bases. |
| Department of Health and Human Services | Food and Drug Administration | No concerns reported. |
| | National Institutes of Health | Agency faces challenges recruiting veterinarians that specialize in labor-atory animal medicine and veterinary pathology, who make up the majority of veterinary positions at the agency. Both specialities are reporting signi-fycant shortages that are not forecast to improve for at least 10 years, whi-ch will hinder the agency's ability to recruit qualified veterinarians. |
| | Centers for Disease Control and Prevention | Veterinarian expertise in agriculture and animal health contribute signify-cantly to human health programs and could be enhanced. |

**Table 1. (Continued)**

| Department | Component agency/other federal entity | Examples of concerns reported by component agency/other federal entity |
|---|---|---|
| | Office of the Assistant Secretary for Preparedness and Response | The Office reported that more than two full-time veterinarians are needed to help develop effective response programs to public health emergencies. Department officials did not support this statement, but said that veterinarians are integral to its response strategy and their continued engagement is essential. |
| Department of Veterans Affairs | Office of Research and Development | No concerns reported. |
| Department of the Interior | U.S. Geological Survey | Salaries are not competitive with the private sector. The agency faces difficulty hiring veterinarians to address wildlife diseases, including those that kill many animals in a single local outbreak. |
| | U.S. Fish and Wildlife Service | Agency has too few veterinarians to monitor diseases in wildlife, nationally and internationally. |
| | National Park Service | Agency has too few veterinarians to address wildlife diseases and survey outbreaks in the vast park system of 84 million acres. |
| Department of Homeland Security | Office of Health Affairs | Agency has too few veterinarians to effectively develop the capabilities to respond to catastrophic food, agriculture, and veterinary events. |
| | Directorate for Science and Technology | No concerns reported. |
| | Directorate for National Protection and Programs | No concerns reported. |
| Smithsonian | National Zoo | Salaries are not competitive; Ameri-can Veterinary Medical Association-specialty boarded status is necessary to perform responsibilities, but com-pensation for this additional training is not available; too few veterinarians to fully conduct agency wildlife health and surveillance studies. |
| Environmental Protection Agency | | No concerns reported. |

Table 1. (Continued)

| Department | Component agency/other federal entity | Examples of concerns reported by component agency/other federal entity |
|---|---|---|
| U.S. Agency for International Development | Bureaus for Economic Growth, Agriculture and Trade; for Global Health; and for Africa | No concerns reported. |
| Department of Commerce | National Oceanic and Atmospheric Administration | Too few veterinarians available to investigate major or multiple outb-reaks, or single events that kill many animals, when they occur in marine animals. |
| National Aeronautics and Space Administration | Office of the Chief Health and Medical Officer | No concerns reported. |
| Department of Energy | Lawrence Livermore National Laboratory | There is a limited number of veteri-narians with the expertise to develop models and conduct analyses to identify the resources agencies will need to respond to animal disease outbreaks, among other things. |
| Department of Justice | Federal Bureau of Investigation | No concerns reported. |

Source: Agency survey responses and interviews.

These current challenges are likely to worsen because a large number of federal veterinarians are eligible to retire in the near future. These retirements would exacerbate the veterinarian shortage and possibly increase interagency competition. Our analysis found that 697 veterinarians at FSIS, APHIS, ARS, Army, and FDA—27 percent of the combined veterinarian workforce of these agencies—are eligible to retire over the next 3 years. As the shortage grows, agencies across the federal government may experience a situation similar to the competition between FSIS and APHIS, and agencies with higher salaries for veterinarians are likely to gain an advantage. As figure 3 illustrates, mean veterinarian base salaries vary widely across agencies, from just under $70,000 at Interior's National Park Service to just about $122,000 at DHS's Office of Health Affairs. Salaries for individual veterinarians range from $35,000 for those in the residency program at the National Zoo to $205,000 for the highest paid veterinarian at NIH.

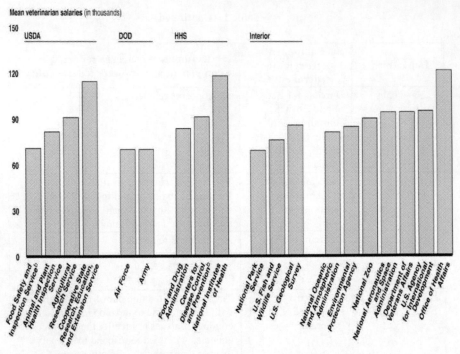

Figure 3. Mean Veterinarian Base Salaries at 19 Component Agencies or Federal Entities in Fiscal Year 2008

Source: GAO analysis of agency data.

Note: Salaries do not include locality pay and stipends. In addition, we do not display mean salary for those agencies with fewer than four veterinarians due to the small number of employees represented. This includes the Departments of Energy and Justice; HHS's Office of the Assistant Secretary for Preparedness and Response; and DHS's Directorate for National Protection and Programs. In addition, DHS's Science and Technology was unable to provide base salary information in time for this report and, therefore, is not included.

[a] We relied on officials from these federal entities to identify mean salaries of all veterinarians employed, including civil and military service employees, contractors, and other, regardless of job title. Because data are means reported by agencies, we could not assess the underlying distribution for outliers or skewness.

[b] This does not include the salaries of the United States Public Health Service Commissioned Corps veterinarians stationed at these agencies. The Commissioned Corps is a uniformed service that belongs to HHS but fills public health leadership and service roles at several federal agencies.

Some agencies, such as those within HHS and the Department of Veterans Affairs, can augment base salaries for veterinarians using special statutory authorities.[7] Agencies can use these authorities to hire veterinarians when standard hiring practices, including the use of recruitment incentives, are impracticable, less effective, or have been exhausted. In addition, DOD can provide all of its veterinarians with a $100 per month stipend, as well as up to an additional $5,000 per year of special pay if they have met the education and training standards of an American Veterinary Medical Association-recognized specialty college.[8] There is no similar authority for USDA veterinarians.

OPM's mission is to ensure the federal government has an effective civilian workforce, but it has not conducted a governmentwide effort to address current and potential veterinarian shortages, as it has done for other professions. For certain professions, OPM has initiated governmentwide direct-hire authority, which allows expediting hiring during a time of critical need or a severe shortage of candidates. For example, in 2003, OPM authorized departments to immediately hire doctors, nurses, and other types of medical professionals without following prescribed competitive procedures. OPM officials told us their agency issued this authority based in part on department and agency concerns. OPM can also hold interagency forums to discuss workforce concerns but has not done so for veterinarians. According to OPM officials, interagency forums are open to all senior human capital representatives from all departments, including USDA and HHS. The forums provide an opportunity to discuss concerns, exchange ideas, and explore solutions to governmentwide staffing issues. OPM officials told us that no department has requested a discussion about veterinarian workforce concerns. Further, officials told us that the agency will facilitate a governmentwide solution, such as an interagency forum, if the departments demonstrate that a shortage exists. Our prior work has identified the need for OPM to use its leadership position to provide assistance to departments and agencies efforts to recruit and retain a capable and committed workforce.[9]

OPM officials told us the agency has taken some steps that could improve veterinarian recruitment and retention. During the course of our review, OPM created a Personnel Action Team to determine whether a governmentwide direct-hire authority should be granted for all veterinarians. OPM did not provide further details other than to state that a decision is expected in early 2009. In addition, OPM recently changed the federal classification of veterinarians. OPM raised the entry grade level for newly hired veterinarians from GS-9 to GS-11 and expanded the description of the federal veterinarian occupation to include areas of specialization, such as toxicology and pathology. OPM officials believe this will help attract more veterinarians into federal service. Agency officials also told us that they meet periodically with departments to ensure occupation classifications meet department needs. This was the first change of the veterinarian classification in over 20 years and was initiated at USDA's request.

The Congress has taken steps that address the broader, national veterinarian shortage, but its efforts thus far have had minimal impact. The National Veterinary Medical Services Act enacted in 2003, directs the Secretary of Agriculture to carry out a program to help veterinarians repay their school loans when they agree to work in areas of need. Although USDA is responsible for implementing the act, it has been delayed in doing so. USDA's Undersecretary for Research, Education, and Economics testified before the Congress that this was because the Cooperative State Research, Education, and Extension Service (CSREES)—the USDA agency in charge of implementation—does not have experience with complex loan repayment programs. The Congress provided initial funding for the act in fiscal year 2006. In August 2008, CSREES began holding public hearings to solicit stakeholder input. Officials from USDA and veterinary associations told us that the $1.8 million allocated thus far for the program is insufficient and would have minimal impact on the shortage. With veterinary student debt averaging $106,000 upon graduation, $1.8 million would cover about 17 students with loans. Moreover, the program targets veterinarians who already have their degree and may not have the skill set the federal government is seeking. To be effective, officials from professional veterinary associations told us, the program would have to provide guarantees and target students early in veterinary school. The Congress also enacted the Higher Education Opportunity Act in August 2008, which has provisions intended to increase the number of veterinarians in the workforce through a competitive grant program that can increase capacity at veterinary colleges. According to the American Veterinary Medical Association, however, these grants will be capped at $500,000 per school, which will not be enough to increase capacity to meet veterinarian demands.

## End Notes

[1] See GAO, *Older Workers: Federal Agencies Face Challenges, But Have Opportunities to Hire and Retain Experienced Employees*, GAO-08-630T (Washington, D.C.: April 30, 2008).

[2] GAO, *Homeland Security: Much Is Being Done to Protect Agriculture from a Terrorist Attack, but Important Challenges Remain*, GAO-05-214 (Washington, D.C.: Mar. 8, 2005).

[3] USDA, Office of Inspector General, Great Plains Region, *Audit Report: Evaluation of FSIS Management Controls Over Pre-Slaughter Activities,* 24601-0007-KC (Washington, D.C.: November 2008).

[4] GAO, *Humane Methods of Slaughter Act: USDA Has Addressed Some Problems but Still Faces Enforcement Challenges*, GAO-04-247 (Washington, D.C.: Jan. 30, 2004).

[5] FDA Science Board, Subcommittee on Science and Technology, *FDA Science and Mission at Risk,* a special report prepared at the request of the Food and Drug Administration (November 2007).

[6] See GAO-04-39; GAO-03-914.

[7] E.g. 38 U.S.C. § 7405; 42 U.S.C. § 209(f).

[8] 37 U.S.C. § 303.

[9] See GAO-08-762T .

In: Veterinarian Workforce Role in Defense...      ISBN: 978-1-60741-656-2
Editor: Justin C. Bennett                           © 2010 Nova Science Publishers, Inc.

*Chapter 4*

# EFFORTS TO IDENTIFY THE VETERINARIAN WORKFORCE NEEDED DURING A PANDEMIC AND LARGE-SCALE ANIMAL DISEASE OUTBREAK ARE INSUFFICIENT

*United States Government Accountability Office*

Four of the five key agencies we reviewed—APHIS, FSIS, ARS, and FDA—have plans intended to detail how essential functions and services, including those that veterinarians perform, would continue during a pandemic that has the potential to severely reduce the workforce. However, each lacks elements that FEMA considers important for effective planning. The Army is still in the process of getting its plan approved and, therefore, we have not evaluated it. In addition, DHS's efforts to identify the veterinarian workforce needed to address a catastrophic nationwide outbreak of foot-and-mouth disease are based on an unrealistic assumption and limited information.

## AGENCY PLANNING TO ENSURE CONTINUITY OF ESSENTIAL VETERINARY FUNCTIONS DURING A PANDEMIC IS INCOMPLETE

FEMA's pandemic guidance assists agencies in identifying special considerations for maintaining essential functions and services during a pandemic outbreak that may cause absenteeism to reach 40 percent. For example, the guidance directs agencies to identify in their pandemic plans how operations will be sustained until normal business activity can be reconstituted, which may be longer than the 30 days usually planned for other types of emergencies. Agency plans are also to identify the essential functions that must be continued on-site and those that can be conducted from a remote location. They also should take into consideration the need for logistical support, services, and infrastructure that help an agency achieve and maintain essential functions and services. To account for the expected high rate of absenteeism at the peak of a pandemic, FEMA guidance also directs agencies to identify at least three people who can carry out each responsibility and identify how the agency will continue to operate if leadership and essential staff are unavailable. Finally, agencies are directed to test their pandemic plans, including the impacts of reduced staffing on facilities and essential functions and services.

APHIS has developed pandemic plans for its headquarters, regional offices, and three laboratories that employ veterinarians, but these plans are missing elements in FEMA's guidance and are not well-organized. For example, they do not explain how animal care, disease investigation, and other essential functions and services would continue if leadership and essential staff are unavailable. Moreover, pieces of these pandemic plans are spread throughout a large number of documents and are not well linked. For example, APHIS officials provided us with an undated pandemic plan that they told us was an appendix to the headquarters continuity of operations plan. But this continuity of operations plan made no reference to such an appendix, and officials were never able to provide us with a document that made reference to such an appendix. USDA recently hired a new emergency preparedness director to revise APHIS's pandemic plans, among other things. The director told us that APHIS recognizes the importance of easily locating the plans and quickly implementing them in the event of a pandemic, and he acknowledged that the current documents are not an effective plan. APHIS is now combining its plans into one comprehensive document that will cover APHIS headquarters, regional offices, and laboratories. In addition, the director told us the new plan, to be completed by early 2009, will better adhere to FEMA guidance.

FSIS has developed a pandemic plan that addresses many of the elements in FEMA's guidance, but it lacks some crucial details. Importantly, the plan takes into account the work that veterinarians do at private slaughter plants. However, it does not address the logistics of how FSIS will work with industry to ensure veterinarians and other employees are available in the event of a pandemic so that food production can continue. FSIS officials told us that they have discussed this logistic with industry and expect, based on these discussions, that some plants would not be able to operate during a pandemic, as a result of FSIS or plant personnel absenteeism. The agency would maintain close communication with industry during a pandemic in order to determine how best to allocate available veterinarians and other FSIS inspection personnel so that slaughter plants could continue to operate. Veterinarians would be allocated to plants based on considerations such as the location of the outbreak and the type of slaughter plant affected. For instance, poultry plants may receive priority consideration because birds can only be slaughtered at a very specific weight. That is, the equipment for processing birds is designed for birds of a very specific size, and industry would not be able to process them if they were permitted to grow too large. However, such logisitcs are absent from FSIS's plan, effectively postponing any decisions until the middle of a crisis. Similarly, the plan does not mention how FSIS would work with APHIS, even though the agencies have formally agreed to jointly plan for critical activities related to surveillance of animal diseases. In addition, the plan does not consider the impact of local quarantines on access to plants.

ARS has developed pandemic plans for all of its 12 laboratories where veterinarians work. We reviewed plans for the two laboratories that employ the most veterinarians: the Southeast Poultry Research Laboratory and the National Animal Disease Center (NADC). These plans are important because they spell out the site-specific details needed to ensure that essential functions at each laboratory can continue. However, the plans lack crucial details, such as how the laboratories will continue operations if absenteeism reaches 40 percent. Specifically, neither of the plans take into account how the laboratories would continue to conduct essential functions and services if leadership and essential staff are unavailable. Agency officials told us they would temporarily suspend projects to account for increased absenteeism, but there is no mention of this in the plans; nor is there mention of how the agency will select projects for suspension or what would trigger suspension. Ensuring a sufficient veterinarian workforce at these laboratories during a pandemic is important because veterinarians carry out critical research and must be available to ensure the proper care of research animals. In addition, NADC is part of a USDA research complex that is transitioning to joint ARS and APHIS support services, including veterinary care for research animals. However, ARS and APHIS have yet to jointly plan for continuity of operations for any type of emergency.

FDA has also developed a pandemic plan, but it is high-level plan that does not address several of FEMA's elements, leaving it unclear if consideration has been given to how veterinarians would carry out any essential functions and services during a pandemic. For example, it does not identify which essential functions—whether they be the responsibility of the veterinarian or others—must be performed on-site and which can be performed remotely. Nor does it explain how veterinarians, or others, will continue operations if absenteeism reaches 40 percent by, for example, delegating authority to three individuals capable of carrying out each of the agency's essential functions. The plan omits other important details, such as contact information for individuals who could assume authority should essential staff and leadership become unavailable. FDA officials told us they will take these gaps into consideration when they update their plan in 2009.

The Army is still in the process of getting its pandemic plan approved and, therefore, we have not evaluated it. According to Army officials, the agency has developed a pandemic plan that has been validated by the U.S. Army Northern Command, but it has not yet been formally referred for approval to the Army's senior leadership, and it does not contain details of how essential functions would continue. According to DOD officials, subordinate divisions within the Army intend to develop detailed plans, but the division responsible for veterinary services (Veterinary Command) has yet to do so. However, DOD officials told us that the Army has been instrumental in helping the United States plan for an outbreak of highly pathogenic avian influenza in birds. Controlling the outbreak in birds reduces the opportunity for the virus to mutate into a strain that could cause a pandemic in humans.

FEMA guidance also directs agencies to test how well their pandemic plans might maintain essential functions and services given reduced staffing levels. FSIS and FDA are the only agencies we reviewed that have done so. In March 2007, FSIS conducted a "tabletop" pandemic exercise where key personnel discuss simulated scenarios in an informal setting in order to test their plans, policies, and procedures. In a summary report, FSIS officials noted that, among other things, additional exercises were needed to improve coordination with industry. FSIS subsequently conducted a similar tabletop exercise with industry in November 2008, but the summary report on lessons learned has yet to be published. FDA conducted an operational exercise in October 2008—a drill to test how well it could continue operations under a staffing shortage. As part of this exercise, FDA tested its ability to reassign tasks, but it is not clear if tasks performed by veterinarians were among those reassigned. FDA officials told us that they plan to issue a report with lessons learned from the exercise in early 2009 and will incorporate that information into FDA's pandemic plan. ARS and APHIS have not tested their plans to see how well their agencies might maintain essential functions and services in the event of reduced staffing levels, but officials told us they intend to do so.

## AN INFEASIBLE ASSUMPTION AND LIMITED INFORMATION HINDER VETERINARIAN WORKFORCE PLANNING EFFORTS FOR A CATASTROPHIC OUTBREAK OF FOOT-AND-MOUTH DISEASE

DHS has two efforts under way that involve identifying the veterinarian workforce needed to quickly perform rapid diagnoses and other essential activities during a large-scale outbreak of foot-and-mouth disease, but both efforts have shortcomings. The first is a long-term national effort that DHS is coordinating to assess the nation's preparedness for multiple, intentional introductions of foot-and-mouth disease. This effort includes identifying the veterinarian workforce and other capabilities that would be needed to best respond to such an outbreak. For example, it has identified the need for 750 veterinarians nationwide to conduct animal health epidemiological investigations and surveillance. It has also identified the need for teams of six livestock and six companion animal veterinarians in each affected state and local jurisdiction to implement disease containment measures, provide animal welfare, and euthanize and dispose of animals.

However, this effort is based on a national planning scenario that USDA and DHS officials' say includes an infeasible assumption. The scenario, developed by a White House Homeland Security Council working group in 2006, involves the mass slaughter of all potentially exposed animals. This "stamping out" method is the same one the United States has used in the past for eradicating smaller outbreaks of foreign animal diseases, but under this scenario, it would result in the slaughter of almost half the nation's beef, dairy, and swine. DHS and USDA officials, as well as state officials who have conducted large-scale foot-and-mouth disease exercises, consider this stamping out method infeasible because, among other things, it would lead to serious logistical and environmental concerns, would not be tolerated by the public, and could wipe out a viable livestock industry. As a result, DHS and USDA officials told us, any workforce estimates produced from this effort are not relevant. However, these officials told us it has helped them better understand the enormity of the workforce response and the coordination that would be required for such a catastrophic event.

DHS and USDA officials told us that to arrive at more relevant workforce estimates, the United States would have to consider alternatives to stamping out for outbreaks as large as the one depicted in the national planning scenario. For example, some countries protect against and control foot-and-mouth disease using vaccines. There are numerous reasons the United States has not used this approach, including limitations to vaccine technology.[1] However USDA, DHS, and state officials recognize that newer, more promising vaccines may play an important role in controlling a catastrophic outbreak. DHS officials also told us that they are looking into revising the Homeland Security Council's planning scenario to make it a more useful planning tool.

For its second effort to identify the veterinarian workforce needed during a foot-and-mouth disease outbreak, DHS has contracted with the Department of Energy's Lawrence Livermore National Laboratory to create a decision support system that models various foot-and-mouth disease outbreak scenarios. This effort includes estimating the number and type of workforce needed for responding to outbreaks, both with and without vaccination. However, according to the project leader, modeling efforts could be improved if certain information were available. For example, in order to model workforce needs for a response that includes the use of vaccines without subsequent stamping out, known as "vaccinate to live," it is important to know what segments of the livestock industry might use such a strategy, and under what circumstances, and how animals and animal products would be identified and their movement tracked. Because the concept of vaccinate to live is new in the United States, USDA has yet to detail in contingency response plans how it would employ this concept, according to agency officials. In the absence of such plans, the project leader, a veterinarian who took part in the response to the 2001 United Kingdom foot-and-mouth disease outbreak, told us that she is left to base her modeling assumptions on personal knowledge and experience, as well as conversations with agency subject matter experts.

Moreover, data limitations make it difficult for any computer modeling effort to accurately predict the spread of the disease. Specifically, modelers must estimate the number and location of animals, as well as their interaction with other segments of industry, because the United States does not have a mandatory, national system that identifies the location and tracks the movement of livestock.[2] Instead, modelers currently use outdated county-level data from USDA's National Agricultural Statistical Survey census, reducing the accuracy of predictions about the spread of foot-and-mouth disease. Also, without knowing the exact location of livestock, it is difficult to understand the interaction between livestock and wildlife. Limited data and information on the number and movement of wildlife and the susceptibility of wildlife populations to the virus further complicates matters, according to agency officials. This is an important gap, since foot-and-mouth disease has been known to spread from livestock to wildlife in past outbreaks. In fact, the last time the United States had an outbreak was in California in the 1920s, when the virus spread from pigs to cattle and black-tailed deer. It took 2 years and the slaughter of 22,000 deer to eradicate the disease from a local deer population in one national park. In areas where livestock graze extensively, there is potential for interaction with susceptible species, such as deer and feral pigs. According to the project leader, as well as USDA and DHS officials, control and eradication strategies would be greatly complicated if wildlife became infected and could require more veterinarians and different expertise. Given the important role wildlife can play in disease outbreak, officials agree it is important to better understand the interaction between livestock and wildlife. In fact, new technologies, such as global positioning systems, have been developed that can, for example, help determine the number and movement of animals, making it possible to gather this type of data, according to a USDA Wildlife Services official. A DHS official told us that, as a first step, it would be important for those agencies with responsibility for overseeing the health of humans, wildlife, and livestock to discuss how wildlife data can be gathered to most accurately model the spread of disease in wildlife.

# End Notes

[1] For more information on why the United States has not used vaccines, see GAO-05-214 .

[2] To understand the issues and our recommendations for helping the United States implement an animal identification system, see GAO, *National Animal Identification System: USDA Needs to Resolve Several Key Implementation Issues to Achieve Rapid and Effective Disease Traceback*, GAO-07-592 (Washington, D.C.: July 6, 2007).

In: Veterinarian Workforce Role in Defense...    ISBN: 978-1-60741-656-2
Editor: Justin C. Bennett                        © 2010 Nova Science Publishers, Inc.

*Chapter 5*

# FEDERAL AND STATE AGENCIES ARE MISSING IMPORTANT OPPORTUNITIES TO ENSURE EFFICIENT USE OF VETERINARIANS DURING DISEASE OUTBREAKS

## *United States Government Accountability Office*

During four recent zoonotic disease outbreaks, the veterinarian workforce challenge cited most often by federal and state officials was having too few veterinarians to control the outbreak while also adequately carrying out other routine activities. Specifically, officials from 3 of 4 federal agencies—APHIS, CDC, and Interior's U.S. Geological Survey (USGS)—and 9 of 13 state agencies cited this challenge. See table 2 for the 17 agencies that were identified as playing an important role, those that cited insufficient veterinarian capacity as a challenge, and other details about these outbreaks.

Two primary reasons emerged for this insufficient capacity. First, according to federal and state officials, veterinarian capacity was insufficient because most of the agencies involved in the four outbreaks had difficulty recruiting and retaining veterinarians in general. For example, officials at many of the public health agencies and diagnostic laboratories we spoke with said that it has been challenging to hire or retain veterinarians with the specialized qualifications they need—public health and pathology skills, respectively. According to 2008 survey results from the American Association of Veterinary Laboratory Diagnosticians, it takes most diagnostic laboratories more than 6 months to fill vacancies for veterinary pathologists. In addition, numerous state agency officials told us that the salaries they offer are not competitive with those of the federal or private sectors. Moreover, officials told us that it has been particularly challenging recruiting veterinarians to work in remote areas or in areas with a high cost of living.

Second, in 2002 and 2003 many veterinarians went to California to address a particularly demanding outbreak of exotic Newcastle disease, limiting the number of veterinarians available to respond to other outbreaks. The exotic Newcastle disease outbreak quickly exhausted California's supply of veterinarians, both at state agencies and APHIS, because so many backyard birds—which are kept as a hobby or for personal consumption—were affected. Responders had to spend valuable time going door-to-door trying to locate potentially infected birds in densely populated urban areas. APHIS called in over 1,000 federal, state, and private-sector veterinarians from outside California to help with the response. But, even with a task force of over 6,000, it took almost a year to control the outbreak. Moreover, because so many veterinarians converged on California, the number available to work on the other three outbreaks—located in Michigan, Wisconsin, and Colorado—was insufficient, according to federal and state agency officials. In part because of the strain on veterinarian resources during the four outbreaks, officials from 16 federal and state agencies expressed concern that they will not have sufficient veterinarian capacity for multiple outbreaks in the future. FDA assisted in one of the four outbreaks and was the only agency not to express concerns about veterinarian capacity. Some federal officials said that the United States has never been tested with two major outbreaks occurring at once, such as simultaneous outbreaks of foot-and-mouth disease and highly pathogenic avian influenza—two highly infectious foreign animal diseases. They said that should this happen, the effects on animal and public health could be devastating.

Federal and state agency officials reported several consequences of this insufficient veterinarian capacity. Examples are as follows:

- Michigan state agency officials told us they had trouble testing enough cattle during the bovine tuberculosis outbreak. Over a 6-1/2 year period, veterinarians struggled to test more than a million cows—an average of more than 3,500 a week—but the state has yet to eradicate the disease.

**Table 2. Four Recent Zoonotic Outbreaks We Analyzed**

| Disease | Location | Date outbreak began | Date outbreak ended | Animals infected | Number of human cases in the identified location | Number of veterinarians involved in outbreak[a] | Total size of workforce involved in outbreak[a] | Federal and state agencies involved in outbreak (agencies in bold cited insufficient veterinarian capacity as a challenge)[b] |
|---|---|---|---|---|---|---|---|---|
| Bovine tuberculosis | Michigan | Fall 1994 | Outbreak is ongoing | Wildlife, cattle | 2[c] | 218[d] | 412 | APHIS<br>**Michigan Department of Agriculture**<br>Michigan Department of Community Health<br>Michigan Department of Natural Resources<br>Michigan State University |
| Exotic Newcastle disease | California | October 2002 | September 2003 | Poultry and other susceptible avian species | 2[c] | 1,250[d] | 6,039 | APHIS<br>California Animal Health and Food Safety Laboratory California Department of Food and Agriculture<br>California Department of Public Health |

**Table 2. (Continued)**

| Disease | Location | Date outbreak began | Date outbreak ended | Animals infected | Number of human cases in the identified location[c] | Number of veterinarians involved in outbreak[a] | Total size of workforce involved in outbreak[a] | Federal and state agencies involved in outbreak (agencies in bold cited insufficient veterinarian capacity as a challenge)[b] |
|---|---|---|---|---|---|---|---|---|
| Monkeypox | Wisconsin | May 2003 | August 2003 | Prairie dogs, Gambian giant rats, dormice, rope squirrels | 27[c] | 39 | 560 | APHIS, CDC, FDA **USGS Wisconsin Dept. of Agriculture, Trade and Consumer Protection Wisconsin Div of Public Health** |
| West Nile virus | Colorado | June 2003 | November 2003[e] | Birds, horses | 2,947[f] | 27 | 150 | APHIS CDC Colorado Department of Agriculture Colorado Department of Public Health and the Environment Colorado Division of Wildlife. Colorado State University |

Source: GAO.

[a] Estimates provided by agency officials. Includes veterinarians across agencies.

[b] The agencies listed are those identified as playing an important role in the outbreak, although additional agencies were involved.

[c] Number of confirmed human cases, as provided by state departments of public health.

[d] These estimates include private-sector veterinarians who worked on the outbreaks as contractors or temporary employees.

[e] West Nile virus is endemic to the United States. There have been seasonal outbreaks across the country every year since 1999.

[f] Number of CDC confirmed human cases. CDC also reports that the number of confirmed nationwide human cases in 2003 for monkeypox and West Nile virus was 51 and 9,862, respectively.

- Some Michigan officials told us that APHIS and the Michigan Department of Agriculture did not have enough veterinarians to both respond to bovine tuberculosis and address other animal diseases, such as *E. coli*. In fact, during all four outbreaks, veterinarians at some point had to delay important work on other diseases, in part because there were not enough veterinarians.[1]
- During the 2003 West Nile virus outbreak in Colorado, a lack of sufficient veterinarians to track and control the disease, among other things, may have allowed the virus to infect more people and animals than it otherwise would have.[2]
- The volume of work required to control and eventually eradicate exotic Newcastle disease in California physically and emotionally exhausted veterinarians to the extent that, once the outbreak was over, they needed significant time off to recover, further delaying work on routine activities.
- The demanding nature of the exotic Newcastle disease and bovine tuberculosis outbreaks may have caused some veterinarians to seek employment elsewhere.

Despite reports of insufficient veterinarian capacity during these four outbreaks, the agencies have not taken full advantage of two important opportunities to learn from past experience. First, 10 of the 17 agencies have not assessed how well their own veterinarian workforces responded to individual outbreaks. Our prior work has shown that agencies can improve response by conducting postoutbreak assessments.[3] One outcome of such an assessment might be a better understanding of how to most efficiently use veterinarians. For example, APHIS—one of the agencies that has performed postoutbreak assessments—found that it had difficulty locating veterinarians with the specialized expertise needed for addressing the exotic Newcastle disease outbreak. As a result, APHIS is developing a national list identifying veterinarians and their credentials to call upon in the future. In addition, federal and state agencies working on bovine tuberculosis in Michigan meet periodically to assess what strategies are working and what they need to change in order to better control the disease. APHIS also conducts periodic reviews of its efforts and the state's efforts to address bovine tuberculosis.

Moreover, none of the 17 agencies have come together to share their experiences across the outbreaks in order to identify workforce challenges that they may have had in common, including veterinarian workforce challenges.

Consequently, the agencies are missing the opportunity to identify and address challenges they are likely to face in the future. The majority of the federal and state agency officials we spoke with agreed that it would be useful for agencies not only to conduct assessments of their own workforce response but also to periodically meet to identify common workforce challenges across multiple outbreaks and discuss strategies for overcoming these challenges. However, some agencies told us that their veterinarian workforce is already facing heavy workload demands that make it difficult for them to meet their existing responsibilities, and thus they have not had time to conduct postoutbreak assessments.

## BOVINE TUBERCULOSIS

Bovine tuberculosis is a contagious disease that can be transmitted from livestock to humans and all other warm-blooded vertebrates. It is a chronic disease, and symptoms are often not apparent until it has reached an advanced stage. Inhalation is the most common route of infection for farm and ranch workers and veterinarians who work with diseased livestock. Calves, hogs, and humans can also contract bovine tuberculosis when they drink unpasteurized milk from infected cows. Livestock are more likely to infect each other when they share a common watering place. The disease's presence in humans has been reduced as a result of a national eradication program, advances in sanitation and hygiene, the discovery of effective drugs, and pasteurization of milk.

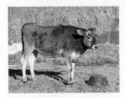

Source: USDA.

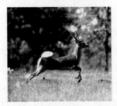

Source: USDA.

## EXOTIC NEWCASTLE DISEASE

Exotic Newcastle disease is caused by a highly contagious virus affecting birds of all species. The virus is spread primarily through direct contact with birds and their bodily discharges. It can also be transmitted through contact with certain objects contaminated with the disease such as vehicles, equipment, shoes, and clothing. It spreads rapidly among birds kept in confinement, such as commercially raised chickens. Many birds die without showing any signs of the disease; however, there are symptoms including, among other things, nasal discharge, coughing, depression, drop in egg production, and swelling around the eyes and neck. Exotic Newcastle disease is only mildly zoonotic in humans, with conjunctivitis being the most common symptom. Other human symptoms include headache, discomfort, and slight chills.

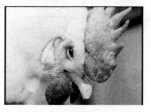

Source: USDA.

## MONKEYPOX

Monkeypox is a rare viral disease that first appeared in the United States in 2003 when a shipment of exotic, wild animals from Ghana, including infected Gambian rats, dormice, and rope squirrels, entered the country. The infected animals then transmitted the virus to prairie dogs when they were collocated at an animal distributor. The prairie dogs were later sold as exotic pets and, in turn, transmitted the disease to humans. People can get monkeypox through a bite or direct contact with the infected animal's blood, body fluids, or lesions. It is thought to be spread person-to-person through large respiratory droplets during direct and prolonged face-to-face contact. In addition, monkeypox can be spread by direct contact with body fluids of an infected person or with virus-contaminated objects, such as bedding or clothing. In humans, the signs and symptoms of monkeypox are similar to those of smallpox and include rash, fever, headache, muscle aches, backache, swollen lymph nodes, a general feeling of discomfort, and exhaustion.

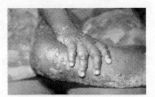

Source: CDC.

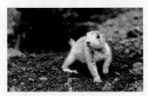

Source: U.S. Fish and Wildlife Service.

## WEST NILE VIRUS

West Nile virus was recently introduced in wild birds and poses a potentially serious threat to people and horses. The virus spread quickly across the United States between 1999 and 2003. Experts believe it is now established as a seasonal epidemic in North America, flaring up in the summer and continuing into the fall. The virus is most often spread when mosquitoes bite infected birds (such as house sparrows or robins), acquire the virus, and then pass it on to other animals or to humans. However, West Nile virus is fatal to many species of wild birds, such as crows, which are then only minimally involved in the spread of the infection. Many people infected with the virus do not become ill. Some experience mild symptoms, including fever, headache, body aches, nausea, vomiting, swollen lymph nodes, or a skin rash. About 1 in 150 develop severe illness and have symptoms that include high fever, headaches, neck stiffness, stupor, disorientation, coma, tremors, convulsions, muscle weakness, vision loss, numbness, and paralysis.

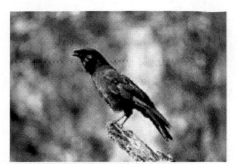

Source: U.S. Fish and Wildlife Service.

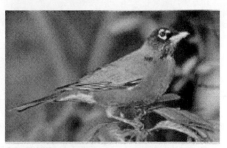

Source: U.S. Fish and Wildlife Service.

## End Notes

[1] Insufficient laboratory resources also affected veterinarians' and other responders' abilities to control outbreaks in a timely manner, according to numerous federal and state agency officials.

[2] CDC officials told us that additional veterinarians may have been beneficial in getting more horses vaccinated. In addition, they said difficulties implementing effective mosquito control programs and getting residents to adopt effective personal protection could also have contributed to a higher number of animal and human infections.

[3] See GAO-06-467T.

In: Veterinarian Workforce Role in Defense...      ISBN: 978-1-60741-656-2
Editor: Justin C. Bennett                      © 2010 Nova Science Publishers, Inc.

*Chapter 6*

# CONCLUSIONS

## *United States Government Accountability Office*

Veterinarians are a small but vital part of the federal workforce, playing important roles in protecting people from zoonotic and foodborne diseases, ensuring the health and humane treatment of food animals, and helping to keep America's food system safe. The nation is facing a growing shortage of veterinarians, and component agencies and other federal entities have already identified insufficiencies in their veterinarian workforces. At FSIS, for example, the veterinarian workforce is finding it difficult to adequately carry out its responsibilities for ensuring food safety and the humane treatment of animals. In 2004, we recommended that FSIS periodically assess whether it has enough inspection resources, including veterinarians, dedicated to humane handling and slaughter activities, but the agency has yet to demonstrate that they have done so. Nor has the federal government conducted the broader assessments and planning activities necessary to address veterinarian workforce problems at FSIS and beyond. Unless USDA and HHS conduct departmentwide assessments of their veterinarian workforces, they will not fully understand the size and nature of the challenges they face in recruiting and retaining veterinarians with the appropriate skills. This will leave their component agencies without a high-level solution to problems they have so far been unable to solve on their own. Moreover, without a governmentwide effort to identify shortcomings in veterinarian capabilities, the federal government may be missing opportunities to find common solutions for attracting veterinarians into federal service.

In addition, unless component agencies complete and test their pandemic plans in keeping with FEMA guidance, they will not be fully prepared to carry out essential veterinarian functions in the face of high rates of absenteeism. Until USDA details how responders would control a foot-and-mouth disease outbreak using vaccines, the nation will not have a complete understanding of the veterinarian workforce needed to control such an outbreak. Similarly, until more information is gathered on the spread of foot-and-mouth disease in wildlife, agencies will not be able to more accurately model the number and type of veterinarians that would be needed if the disease were to spread beyond livestock. Failure to understand the workforce needed during a catastrophic event—whether a pandemic or an attack on the food supply— could unnecessarily increase the scope and severity of the crisis. Finally, unless component agencies involved in responding to outbreaks of zoonotic disease regularly review their own performance and collectively assess opportunities for improvement, they cannot be assured they are using veterinarians as efficiently as possible. They are, therefore, more likely to face an insufficient veterinarian workforce capacity during future outbreaks, which may cause an unnecessary increase in the severity of the outbreaks and worsen the threat to public health.

In: Veterinarian Workforce Role in Defense...    ISBN: 978-1-60741-656-2
Editor: Justin C. Bennett                © 2010 Nova Science Publishers, Inc.

*Chapter 7*

# RECOMMENDATIONS FOR EXECUTIVE ACTION

## *United States Government Accountability Office*

We are making nine recommendations to improve the ability of the federal veterinarian workforce to carry out routine activities, prepare for a catastrophic event, and respond to zoonotic disease outbreaks.

To help ensure the federal veterinarian workforce is sufficient to meet the critical responsibilities it carries out on a routine basis, we recommend that

1. the Secretary of Agriculture direct FSIS to periodically assess whether its level of inspection resources dedicated to food safety and humane slaughter activities is sufficient, and

2. the Secretary of Agriculture conduct a departmentwide assessment of USDA's veterinarian workforce—based, for example, on workforce assessments by its component agencies—to identify current and future workforce needs (including training and employee development) and departmentwide solutions to problems shared by its agencies. When the Secretary completes the assessment, the results should be forwarded to the Director of the Office of Personnel Management.

3. We also recommend that the Secretary of Health and Human Services direct the department's component agencies that employ veterinarians to conduct regular workforce assessments and that the Secretary then conduct a departmentwide assessment of HHS's veterinarian workforce to identify current and future workforce needs (including training and employee development) and solutions to problems shared by its agencies. When the Secretary completes the assessment, the results should be forwarded to the Director of the Office of Personnel Management.

4. Finally, we recommend that the Director of the Office of Personnel Management determine, based on USDA's and HHS's departmentwide veterinarian workforce evaluations, whether a governmentwide effort is needed to address shortcomings in the sufficiency of the current and future veterinarian workforce.

To help the veterinarian workforce continue essential functions during a pandemic, we recommend that

5. the Secretaries of Agriculture, Defense, and Health and Human Services ensure that their component agencies that employ veterinarians complete pandemic plans that contain the necessary elements put forth in DHS's continuity of operations pandemic guidance, including periodically testing, training, and exercising plans.

To improve estimates of the veterinarian workforce needed to respond to a large-scale foot-and-mouth disease outbreak, we recommend that

6. the Secretary of Agriculture detail in a contingency response plan how a response using vaccines would be implemented, and

7. the Secretary of Homeland Security coordinate an interagency effort to identify the data necessary to model the spread of disease in wildlife and how best to gather these data.

To improve the ability of the federal veterinarian workforce to respond to zoonotic outbreaks in the future while also effectively carrying out routine activities, we recommend that the Secretaries of those departments most likely

to be involved in response efforts—such as USDA, HHS, and Interior—ens
that their agencies:

8. conduct postoutbreak assessments of workforce management; and

9. in coordination with relevant federal, state, and local agencies, periodically review the postoutbreak assessments to identify common workforce challenges and strategies for addressing them.

In: Veterinarian Workforce Role in Defense...    ISBN: 978-1-60741-656-2
Editor: Justin C. Bennett    © 2010 Nova Science Publishers, Inc.

*Chapter 8*

# AGENCY COMMENTS AND OUR EVALUATION

## *United States Government Accountability Office*

We provided a draft of this report to USDA, DOD, HHS, OPM, DHS, and Interior for their review and comment. USDA, DOD, OPM, DHS, and Interior generally agreed with the recommendations. HHS generally concurred with the report but not with one finding we reported regarding FDA's veterinarian workforce. Also, all departments provided technical comments, which we incorporated as appropriate.

USDA agreed that it should periodically assess whether its level of inspection resources dedicated to food safety and humane slaughter activities is sufficient and believes that FSIS is already doing this assessment as a part of its budget formulation process. However, we made this recommendation in 2004, and are repeating it now, because FSIS has yet to demonstrate that they have done this assessment. USDA also reported that because APHIS and FSIS employ the majority of veterinarians within the department, these component agencies will work together, with departmental consultation, as needed, to develop solutions to shared problems. We continue to believe that a departmentwide assessment is necessary. In addition, the department commented that it will track veterinarian workforce trends and devise strategies to train, recruit, and retain veterinarians in order to mitigate attrition and maintain progress toward the department's mission to protect the public health. Furthermore, USDA reported that APHIS and FSIS are already taking steps to revise their pandemic plans to overcome many of the gaps we identified to help ensure the USDA veterinarian workforce can carry out essential functions during a pandemic. USDA's written comments and our evaluation appear in appendix III.

DOD stated that efforts are under way to finalize the Army's pandemic influenza plan and that the implementation date will be determined based on current mission priorities. DOD's written comments and our evaluation appear in appendix IV.

HHS reported that veterinarians are essential to protecting the health of the American people. In addition, the department commented that veterinarians are a valuable resource at CDC and conducting workforce assessments, as recommended in our report, will ensure that HHS maintains a sufficient capacity for outbreak response. HHS further reported that all operating staff division heads are required to have workforce plans in place for their organizations by September 2009. Once the plans are completed, the HHS Office of Human Resources will look across the plans to identify opportunities for collaboration with regard to strategic recruitment, development, and retention. The department also plans to strengthen its oversight of the operating divisions to ensure that they are implementing their workforce plans, focusing on those occupations critical to the success of their missions. While veterinarians are not currently identified as a department-level Mission Critical Occupation, largely because they represent less than 1 percent of the HHS workforce, the department plans to review its Mission Critical Occupations in the coming year using criteria that are more risk-based. However, HHS did not agree with a statement in our report that references a 2007 FDA Advisory Committee report claiming that CVM is in a state of crisis. The department stated that, given the broad nature of the 2007 Advisory Committee report, it is not applicable to veterinarians. However, we reported information pertaining directly to vetcrinarians—information we obtained from an interview with an author of the Advisory Committee report. Furthermore, HHS stated that CVM has made great strides in the past few years assessing its workforce needs and that the 2007 report is outdated. Our report identifies many of the efforts CVM has recently undertaken, such as hiring additional veterinarians and beginning an effort to analyze the gap between current resources and needs. It also notes that, according to FDA officials, the agency is undertaking significant reforms to address fundamental concerns in the 2007 report. However, as our report also states, FDA did not tell us how these efforts address the identified veterinarian skill gap specifically. HHS's written comments and our evaluation appear in appendix V.

OPM informed us that it has established a team to research and analyze data to determine the feasibility of issuing a governmentwide direct-hire authority for veterinarians under its statutory and regulatory authority. OPM did not provide further details except to say that a decision is expected early in 2009. Until this study is completed, OPM relies on individual agencies to make such requests when they have encountered a severe shortage of candidates or a critical hiring need for veterinarians. In addition, OPM informed us that on November 25, 2008, it approved USDA's request for direct-hire authority. OPM also commented that, in 2003, the agency approved direct-hire authority for temporary and term positions, including veterinarians, to help protect the health or safety of the U.S. food supply during a pandemic or other declared emergency situation. OPM's written comments and our evaluation appear in appendix VI.

DHS recommended that the federal government enhance efforts to identify the veterinarian workforce needed during catastrophic events. They stated that this could be achieved through an OPM pursuit of a multidepartment assessment of veterinary manpower requirements. They further recommended that agencies develop plans that identify how veterinarians will continue essential functions during additional catastrophic events, taking into consideration the potential for absenteeism that exceeds the level of 40 percent estimated for a pandemic. In addition, DHS stated that, once a governmentwide veterinarian workforce need is determined, effective recruitment and retention programs should be developed that are consistent across all agencies. However, DHS disagreed with our finding that the estimate produced from one of its efforts to identify the workforce needed during a catastrophic outbreak of foot-and-mouth disease is not relevant. We continue to believe, as does DHS, that this effort is based on an infeasible assumption. Therefore, we do not agree that this estimate is relevant to any response that could reasonably be implemented during such an outbreak. DHS's written comments and our evaluation appear in appendix VII.

Interior commended GAO for conducting a well-researched examination of the federal veterinarian workforce. The department emphasized the importance of including wildlife disease expertise in a strategy for protecting human and animal health. The department also identified the importance of detecting and preventing non-native invasive infectious diseases from entering U.S. borders via imported wildlife as important to protecting human and animal health. Interior's written comments and our evaluation appear in appendix VIII.

As agreed with your offices, unless you publicly announce the contents of this report earlier, we plan no further distribution until 22 days from the report date. At that time, we will send copies to the Secretaries of Agriculture, Commerce, Defense, Energy, Health and Human Services, Homeland Security, Interior, Justice, Smithsonian Institution, and Veterans Affairs; the Director of the Office of Personnel Management; the Administrators of the Environmental Protection Agency, National Aeronautics and Space Administration, and U.S. Agency for International Development; appropriate congressional committees; and other interested parties. The report also will be available at no charge on the GAO Web site at http://www.gao.gov.

If you or your staff have any questions about this report, please contact me at (202) 512-3841 or shamesl@gao.gov. Contact points for our Offices of Congressional Relations and Public Affairs may be found on the last page of this report. GAO staff who made contributions to this report are listed in appendix IX.

Sincerely yours,

Lisa Shames
Director, Natural Resources
and Environment

In: Veterinarian Workforce Role in Defense… ISBN: 978-1-60741-656-2
Editor: Justin C. Bennett © 2010 Nova Science Publishers, Inc.

*Chapter 9*

# APPENDIX I: LOCATION AND RESPONSIBILITIES OF VETERINARIANS IN THE FEDERAL GOVERNMENT

## *United States Government Accountability Office*

| Number of veterinarians by department | Number of veterinarians by component agency or other entity[a] | | | Examples of veterinarian responsibilities |
|---|---|---|---|---|
| Department of Agriculture | 1,771 | Animal and Plant Health Inspection Service | 667 | Protect American livest-ock and poultry health through diagnosis, control and eradication of animal diseases, and partnering with state officials to manage and eradicate disease outbreaks. Some are employed overseas. |
| | | Food Safety and Inspection Service | 1,043[b] | Inspect livestock and pou-ltry at slaughter plants to identify and examine dis-eased animals, and prev-ent their entry into the nation's food supply; det-ermine the significance of disease conditions and their potential hazard to public health; and may oversee total inspection operations. |

**(Continued)**

| Number of veterinarians by department | Number of veterinarians by component agency or other entity[a] | | Examples of veterinarian responsibilities |
|---|---|---|---|
| | Agricultural Research Service | 57 | Conduct critical research to develop solutions for high-priority agricultural problems, such as highly pathogenic avian influenza. |
| | Cooperative State Research, Education, and Extension Service | 4 | Plan, develop, organize, and manage animal health related research, educati-on, and extension progr-ams in coordination with other federal agencies and national and international efforts. |
| Department of Defense | 841 | Army[c] | 753 | Ensure food safety at De-partment of Defense loca-tions; develop medical defenses against chemical and biological warfare threat agents; conduct intelligence work; and care for service animals. |
| | | Air Force | 88 | Track infectious diseases among Air Force person-nel, oversee the health of Air Force personnel for deployment, and ensure food safety at Air Force bases. |
| Department of Health and Human Services[d] | 316 | Food and Drug Administration | 152 | Ensure that animal food and drugs are safe and effective; that food from medically treated animals is safe to eat; and help ensure the safety of food, drugs, and cosmetics, among other things. |
| | | National Institutes of Health | 85 | Support all animal aspects of its intramural research program by providing regulatory oversight of research animals, provi-ding disease surveillance and diagnostics, managing the agency compliance office, and conducting conducting basic scientific and translational research. |

**(Continued)**

| Number of veterinarians by department | Number of veterinarians by component agency or other entity[a] | | Examples of veterinarian responsibilities |
|---|---|---|---|
| | | Centers for Disease Control and Prevention | 77 | Work to identify, prevent, and control public health threats through applied epidemiology, laboratory animal medicine and tox-icology, technical assis-tance and consultation, surveillance, field and clinical investigations, and human-animal interface research; support public health training and active-ities among state, local, tribal, and global health programs; provide expe-rtise in public health emergency preparedness and provide surge capa-city following public health disasters, global disease outbreaks, and terrorist attacks; and prevent importation at ports of entry of animals/ animal products that pose human health risks. |
| | | Office of the Assistant Secretary for Preparedness and Response | 2 | Identifies, coordinates, and provides qualified veteran-ary medical personnel for events requiring emerge-ncy and disaster-related veterinary medical care services to impacted anim-al populations (including household pets and service animals) in or outside of shelter locations until local infrastructures are reestablished. |
| Department of Veterans Affairs | 37 | Office of Research and Development | 37 | Conduct research to imp-rove the health of veteran-ns and oversee the health and welfare of animals used in research. |
| Department of the Interior | 24 | U.S. Geological Survey | 16 | Investigate, diagnose, develop control methods, and develop databases for wildlife diseases; provide training to wildlife biol-ogists and resource managers in wildlife |

## (Continued)

| Number of veterinarians by department | Number of veterinarians by component agency or other entity[a] | | Examples of veterinarian responsibilities |
|---|---|---|---|
| | | | dis-ease identification and control; conduct clinical veterinary research on wildlife diseases; and oversee the health and welfare of experimental and wild animals used in research, including rese-arch on wildlife diseases. |
| | U.S. Fish and Wildlife Service | 4 | Perform fish health mana-gement and diagnostic activities; conduct wildl-ife disease surveillance, diagnostics, and outbreak investigations; provide technical expertise; and draft policy, regulation, and management action plans. |
| | National Park Service | 4 | Prepare surveillance and contingency response pla-ns for addressing import-ant wildlife diseases in the park system; formul-ate policies for manage-ment of wildlife diseases. |
| Department of Homeland Security | 16 Office of Health Affairs | 8 | Provide professional veterinary expertise and leadership to defend human and animal health and the nation's agriculture and food supply against terro-rist attacks, major disasters, and other emergencies. |
| | Directorate for Science and Technology | 6 | Utilize knowledge and skills of disease movement, risk, and economic impacts of diseases to oversee programs regard-ing the safety of U.S. agriculture and food supply. |
| | Directorate for National Protection and Programs | 2 | Identify technologies and capabilities that can be used to help assure the protection of the nation's agriculture and food supp-ly from a terrorist attack. |

## (Continued)

| Number of veterinarians by department | Number of veterinarians by component agency or other entity[a] | | Examples of veterinarian responsibilities |
|---|---|---|---|
| Smithsonian | 16 | National Zoo    16 | Protect the health of endangered species under the auspices of the Natio-nal Zoo and oversee the health of animals housed at the National Zoo; study disease dynamics and pathology of disease in endangered species; cond-uct research in endingered species conservation and propagation, and surveillance and research in emerging diseases of non-domestic animals include-ing wildlife; train veteri-narians and advance vete-rinary medical knowledge regarding zoo and wild animal species in the Uni-ted States and abroad; administer International Veterinary Training program. |
| Environmental Protection Agency | 13 | 13 | Assess the risks of pesticide use to humans and domestic animals, research the cancer risk of environmental chemicals, and improve the process for managing potential environmental carcinogens. |
| U.S. Agency for Interna-tional Develop-ment | 8 | Bureaus for Economic Growth, Agriculture and Trade; for Global Health; and for Africa    8 | Provide guidance on iss-ues related to management of highly pathogenic avian influenza outbreaks and recovery; identify opportunities to share and leverage resources for avian influenza response efforts with international and domestic health agencies and universities. |
| Department of Commerce | 9 | National Oceanic and Atmospheric Administration    9 | Conduct audits of seafood plants and products as part of the Seafood Inspection Program; provide guidelines and oversight of the Marine |

| (Continued) | | | | |
|---|---|---|---|---|
| **National Aeronautics and Space Administration** | **Number of veterinarians by component agency or other entity[a]** | | **Examples of veterinarian responsibilities** | |
| Department of Energy | | | | Mammal Health and Stranding Response Program, Aquatic Animal Health Program, disease surveillance, health monitoring, outbreak investigations, and contaminants/pathogen/toxin/ health research. |
| Department of Justice | 5 | Office of the Chief Health and Medical Officer | 5 | Provide and coordinate animal care at agency research facilities; one veterinarian is an astronaut. |

Source: GAO analysis of agency survey responses and interviews.

[a] We relied on federal agency officials to identify all veterinarians employed—civil and military service employees, contractors, and other—regardless of job title. The number of veterinarians reported for all agencies are as of June 30, 2008, except for the following: The Food Safety Inspection Service (FSIS) and the Army veterinary reserve corps are current as of the end of fiscal year 2008 and November 2008, respectively.

[b] The number of veterinarians listed for FSIS include 968 veterinary medical officers, the majority of whom work at slaughter plants, as well as approximately 75 veterinarians who work in other occupations.

[c] The Army veterinarian workforce consists of 446 active duty; 173 reserve corps; and 134 other.

[d] The number of veterinarians listed for the Department of Health and Human Services does not include those United States Public Health Service Commissioned Corps veterinarians working at the FSIS and the Environmental Protection Agency because they are counted as employees of those agencies.

In: Veterinarian Workforce Role in Defense...        ISBN: 978-1-60741-656-2
Editor: Justin C. Bennett                                © 2010 Nova Science Publishers, Inc.

**Chapter 10**

# APPENDIX II: SCOPE AND METHODOLOGY

## United States Government Accountability Office

To determine the extent to which the federal government has assessed the sufficiency of its veterinarian workforce for routine activities, we interviewed officials and collected documents from the American Veterinary Medical Association, the National Association of Federal Veterinarians (NAFV), and the Association of American Veterinary Medical Colleges to identify general concerns about the federal veterinarian workforce. NAFV also provided a review it had conducted in 1996 that identified federal departments and agencies that employ veterinarians. We expanded this list of departments and component agencies based on referrals and experience from our past reports, resulting in a list of 24 component agencies and other federal entities. We then surveyed these 24 entities to obtain information on the federal veterinarian workforce—including the number of veterinarians employed, their grade level, salaries, roles and responsibilities, number of vacancies, and sufficiency of the workforce. We conducted this self-administered electronic survey in October 2007 and then requested an update of this survey information in July 2008. We achieved a 100 percent response rate both times. However, one entity was unable to provide some of the specific salary information we requested, and we noted this in our report.

Because this was not a sample survey, but rather a survey of the universe of respondents, it has no sampling errors. However, the practical difficulties of conducting any survey may introduce errors, commonly referred to as nonsampling errors. For example, respondents may have difficulty interpreting a particular question, the sources of information available to respondents may introduce errors or variability, and analysts may introduce errors when entering data into a database or analyzing these data. We took steps in developing the questionnaire, collecting the data, and analyzing them to minimize such nonsampling error. For example, we pretested the survey to ensure that the questions were relevant, clearly stated, and easy to understand.

To obtain salary information for Department of Agriculture (USDA) agencies over the past 5 years, we used data from the Office of Personnel Management's (OPM) Central Personnel Data File. We did not independently verify these data for the years we reviewed; however, in a 1998 report, we found that governmentwide data from this file for the key variables in this study (agency, birth date, service computation date, occupation, and retirement plan) were 99 percent accurate or better.[1] Therefore, we feel these data were sufficiently reliable for the purposes of this review.

On the basis of information we received in our survey of these component agencies and other entities, we then analyzed the workforce assessment efforts of USDA, the Department of Defense (DOD), and the Department of Health and Human Services (HHS). We selected these departments because they employ the majority of federal veterinarians (96 percent) identified in our survey. Within these three departments, we further focused our review on five component agencies—the Animal and Plant Health Inspection Service (APHIS), FSIS, Army, and the Food and Drug Administration (FDA)—to determine the extent to which they assessed the sufficiency of their veterinarian workforce. We also selected the Agricultural Research Service (ARS) for further review because it is USDA's chief scientific research agency and conducts research to solve agricultural problems of high national priority. We conducted our assessment by reviewing department and agency documents, such as workforce plans, human capital management reports, workforce models, and gap assessments. We then compared workforce assessment efforts of the three departments and five component agencies with GAO workforce planning guidance. We also conducted semistructured interviews with workforce planning and veterinarian program officials. In addition, we interviewed an author of the report *FDA Science and Mission at Risk* regarding the report's findings and their relation to FDA veterinarian skill gaps. Further, we visited one poultry and two beef slaughter plants of varying sizes to observe conditions and interview veterinarians and other FSIS officials. We also interviewed FSIS officials working at the slaughter plant that was the subject of the nation's largest beef recall. We selected these plants on the basis of proximity to the sites of the four recent zoonotic disease outbreaks we reviewed, and recommendations from FSIS officials. Moreover, other veterinarians contacted us to relay concerns about the sufficiency of the FSIS veterinarian workforce. We interviewed officials from the OPM to determine the agency's role in workforce planning for federal veterinarians and to identify recruitment and retention authorities available to agencies and departments. Finally, we interviewed experts from the Council of State and Territorial Epidemiologists, the National Association of State Public Health Veterinarians, the American College of Veterinary Pathologists, the American Association of Wildlife Veterinarians, the American Association of Veterinary Laboratory Diagnosticians, and the National Academy of Sciences to identify workforce needs for veterinary specialties including public health, wildlife veterinarians, veterinary laboratory diagnostics, and veterinary pathology.

To determine the extent to which the federal government has identified the veterinarian workforce needed during a catastrophic event, we analyzed workforce planning efforts for two potential large-scale national incidents that the White House Homeland Security Council deemed critical for planning purposes: a pandemic and a foot-and-mouth disease outbreak. For the first, we compared pandemic plans from APHIS, FSIS, ARS, Army, and FDA to guidance the Department of Homeland Security's (DHS) Federal Emergency Management Agency provided to departments and agencies for identifying special considerations for maintaining essential functions and services under such conditions.[2,3] These agencies were selected for the reasons described above. We interviewed agency officials to discuss identified gaps and determine the extent to which the plans were being updated and tested. Furthermore, we interviewed HHS officials to understand their review of state pandemic plans, which are under development to ensure continuity of the food supply system and the ability to respond to agriculture emergencies. For the second, we reviewed veterinarian workforce outcomes from DHS's nationwide effort to assess the nation's preparedness for multiple, intentional introductions of foot-and-mouth disease. In addition to interviewing the DHS official responsible for coordinating the animal health emergency capability, we also interviewed state officials who have conducted large-scale exercises simulating a response to foot-and-mouth disease, as well as USDA officials with responsibility for such an event, to determine the feasibility of the response depicted in the scenario. Because vaccine use was suggested as an alternative strategy to the slaughter of animals infected with foot-and-mouth disease, we also interviewed USDA's Chief Veterinary Officer, and DHS and USDA officials at Plum Island Animal Disease Center to determine the status of foot-and-mouth disease vaccine development and the feasibility, as well as practicality, of their use. Finally, at the recommendation of DHS, we interviewed the Department of Energy official responsible for overseeing the development of a decision support system that models various foot-and-mouth disease outbreak scenarios in order to estimate the number and type of workforce needed for responding to outbreaks. The Department of Energy is performing this work under contract for DHS. We also interviewed USDA, DHS, and Department of the Interior (Interior) officials to determine the extent to which agencies are including the possible spread of foot-and-mouth disease in wildlife in their planning efforts.

To determine the extent to which federal and state agencies encountered veterinarian workforce challenges during four recent zoonotic outbreaks, we conducted semistructured interviews with 17 federal and state agencies involved in these outbreaks. We relied on federal and state officials to identify those agencies that played an important role in outbreak response. Based on this information, we then interviewed officials from USDA, HHS, Interior, state public health departments, state agriculture and wildlife agencies, state diagnostic laboratories, and one county public health agency. We also interviewed other individuals involved in the outbreaks, including researchers from Northwestern University, the University of California at Davis, and Western University of Health Sciences. We selected the four outbreaks in our review—bovine tuberculosis in Michigan, exotic Newcastle disease in California, monkeypox in Wisconsin, and West Nile virus in Colorado— because these outbreaks were most frequently recommended by federal officials as examples of recent zoonotic diseases; are ongoing or have occurred since 2001; and have affected various types of animals, including livestock, wildlife, pets, and exotic animals. In addition, we chose these four outbreaks for review because of the unique nature of the outbreaks in these states. Specifically, we selected Michigan as the state for the bovine tuberculosis review because the ongoing outbreak is the longest outbreak of this disease in the United States in recent history. We chose California because it experienced the greatest number of animal infections for the exotic Newcastle disease outbreak. We selected Wisconsin because it experienced the most human monkeypox infections. We selected Colorado for West Nile virus because the number of human infections in Colorado in 2003 was the highest for a single state. In addition to the interviews, we also analyzed federal, state, and county documents, such as after action reports, in order to (1) understand the extent to which agencies formally assessed the management of their veterinarian workforces during these outbreaks and (2) identify any workforce-related challenges and steps agencies took to address these challenges.

## End Notes

[1] GAO, *OPM's Central Personnel Data File: Data Appear Sufficiently Reliable to Meet Most Customer Needs*, GAO/GGD-98-199 (Washington, D.C.: Sept. 30, 1998).

[2] To learn more about federal guidance for pandemic planning, see
http://www.pandemicflu.gov/plan/federal/index.html.

[3] GAO has a separate review under way that is looking at federal agency plans for protecting the workforce while maintaining their essential functions during a pandemic.

In: Veterinarian Workforce Role in Defense...        ISBN: 978-1-60741-656-2
Editor: Justin C. Bennett                      © 2010 Nova Science Publishers, Inc.

**Chapter 11**

# APPENDIX III: COMMENTS FROM THE DEPARTMENT OF AGRICULTURE

## *United States Government Accountability Office*

Note: GAO comments supplementing those in the report text appear at the end of this appendix.

USDA

United States Department of Agriculture

Office of the Secretary
Washington, D.C. 20250

JAN 16 2009

Ms. Lisa Shames
Director
Natural Resources and Environment
United States Government Accountability Office
441 G Street N.W.  Mail Room 2T23A
Washington, DC 20548

Dear Ms. Shames:

Thank you for allowing the United States Department of Agriculture (USDA) the opportunity to comment on the GAO draft report "Veterinarian Workforce: Actions Are Needed to Ensure Sufficient Capacity for Protecting Public and Animal Health" (09-178). We are providing comments to the Recommendations for Executive Action for USDA.

**Recommendation #1**

**To help ensure the federal veterinarian workforce is sufficient to meet the critical responsibilities it carries out on a routine basis, GAO recommends that the Secretary of Agriculture direct FSIS to periodically assess whether its level of inspection resources dedicated to food safety and humane slaughter activities is sufficient.**

USDA agrees with the recommendation and already regularly assesses the level of inspection resources it needs. As part of the budget formulation process, the Food Safety and Inspection Service (FSIS) annually assesses its needs for the inspection and veterinary resources sufficient to meet the statutory mandates for food safety and the humane handling of livestock. Also, as mentioned in the GAO report, FSIS is continually taking steps to enhance veterinary and inspection capacities and to better allocate its resources to protect the public health.

In addition, in the course of operations FSIS managers conduct regular assessments to determine the number of Public Health Veterinarians (PHV) positions needed in specific establishments, primarily by considering the geographic location or proximity of other federal establishments, the size of the establishment, the production volume of plant operations (which determines the number of on-line inspection personnel), and the number of approved operational shifts. Multiple slaughter plants located in close proximity can be assigned a single PHV on a patrol basis while slaughter establishments in more remote locations may require a PHV at each plant. In slaughter plants with extremely high production volume, FSIS may assign an additional PHV.

An Equal Opportunity Employer

See comment 1.      See comment 2.

Ms. Lisa Shames

In addition to the above response, we have further general comments pertaining to GAO's analysis of FSIS operations and activities for publication in the final report. These general comments are contained in the attached appendix.

**Recommendation #2**

**To help ensure the federal veterinarian workforce is sufficient to meet the critical responsibilities it carries out on a routine basis, GAO recommends that the Secretary of Agriculture conduct a departmentwide assessment of USDA's veterinarian workforce—based, for example, on workforce assessments by its component agencies—to identify current and future workforce needs (including training and employee development) and departmentwide solutions to problems shared by its agencies. When USDA completes its assessment, it should forward the results to the Director of OPM.**

USDA agrees with this recommendation. However, given that the majority of USDA's veterinary workforce is located in two agencies--the Animal and Plant Health Inspection Service (APHIS) and FSIS (40 percent and 57 percent, respectively), and that each has both the staff as well as the expertise to conduct the assessments and analyze the data, APHIS and FSIS will conduct veterinary workforce analyses for their respective agencies and work together, with Departmental consultation, as needed, to develop solutions to problems shared by both agencies. Agency-specific problems will be addressed separately within the respective agency. Veterinary workforce trends will be tracked, and training, recruitment and retention strategies devised to mitigate attrition and maintain progress toward the Department's mission to protect the public health. Assessment results will then be forwarded to the Director of OPM.

**Recommendation #5**

**To help the veterinarian workforce continue essential functions during a pandemic, GAO recommends that the Secretaries of Agriculture, Defense and Health and Human Services ensure that their component agencies that employ veterinarians complete pandemic plans that contains the necessary elements put forth in DHS's continuity of operations pandemic guidance, including periodically testing, training, and exercising plans.**

USDA agrees with this recommendation. The active Pandemic Plan (Plan) was written in January 2007 by APHIS. However, that Plan is now currently being updated and modernized based upon the Department of Homeland Security's (DHS) Pandemic Plan checklist that was published in July of 2008. The checklist was developed by DHS to

See comment 3.

Ms. Lisa Shames

assist Departments and Agencies in creating a complete and workable Pandemic Plan based on ensuring that the primary essential functions of an agency, in this case APHIS, will continue to be performed. Included among the provisions of that checklist is the requirement for periodic testing, training and exercising of the Plan. The revised Plan is expected to be ready for internal review, coordination, and collaboration with the regions, programs, and various stakeholders by the end of January 2009 with a final document in place by March 2009.

## Recommendation #6

**To improve estimates of the veterinarian workforce needed to respond to a large-scale foot-and-mouth disease outbreak, GAO recommends that the Secretary of Agriculture detail in a contingency response plan how a response using vaccines would be implemented.**

USDA agrees with this recommendation. USDA has issued contingency plans for use of foot-and-mouth disease (FMD). Specifically, APHIS has issued contingency plans for use of FMD vaccine as a sponsor of the North American Foot-and-Mouth Disease Vaccine Bank (NAFMDVB). The NAFMDVB holds FMD concentrated antigens, which can be finished into vaccine in the event of a FMD outbreak in one of the member countries (United States, Canada and Mexico). In addition, APHIS' Foreign Animal Disease Preparedness and Response Plan includes a decision tree which outlines the decision-making process that would lead to the use of vaccine as an aid in the control and eradication of FMD in North America.

Policy decisions as to who may administer the vaccine will be made based upon the circumstances of the outbreak. If the outbreak is FMD and a vaccination strategy is chosen, multiple options exist. The considerations include activating the National Animal Health Emergency Response Corps; federalizing private veterinarians who have pre-qualified; utilizing the federally accredited veterinarian workforce in addition to regulatory (federal and State) veterinarians; or allowing animal owners to vaccinate, under appropriate veterinary supervision with respect to State laws.

Looking to the future, USDA and DHS are actively supporting the development and application of new vaccine technologies, like molecular based vaccines, that do not require expensive, high-containment production facilities and can be produced safely in the United States.

## Recommendation #8

**To improve the ability of the federal veterinarian workforce to respond to zoonotic outbreaks in the future while also effectively carrying out routine activities, GAO recommends that the secretaries of those departments most likely to be involved in**

Ms. Lisa Shames

response efforts—such as USDA, HHS, and the Interior—ensure that their agencies conduct post-outbreak assessments of workforce management.

USDA agrees with this recommendation. USDA has conducted or commissioned assessments of the response workforce and used findings to direct its response planning. This has generated the development and utilization of a resource ordering and status system, based on the Forest Service tool that allows for real-time management of resources, including trained personnel, to either support the response or maintain regular functions. Internal evaluations of response team deployments and activities have led to a more integrated team approach which will be introduced in 2009. Another approach to adequately address surge needs in a response effort that has been highly successful and merits possible expansion is the utilization of 3D (depopulation, disposal and decontamination) contractors. Companies contracted by APHIS and trained in advance have arrived on-the-scene within 24 hours, freeing veterinarians to work on incident management, surveillance or epidemiological studies.

### Recommendation #9

**To improve the ability of the federal veterinarian workforce to response to zoonotic outbreaks in the future while also effectively carrying out routine activities, GAO recommends that the secretaries of those departments most likely to be involved in response efforts—such as USDA, HHS and the Interior—ensure that their agencies in coordination with relevant federal, state, and local agencies, periodically review the post-outbreak assessments to identify common workforce challenges and strategies for addressing them.**

USDA agrees with this recommendation. Specifically, USDA agrees that commonalities exist among response agencies when faced with an animal or public health emergency that creates immediate needs for trained and ready personnel. We will continue to collaborate with the agencies listed in support of mutual goals, such as the requirements of Homeland Security Presidential Declarations and ensuring a workforce adequate to manage crises.

Sincerely,

Bruce I. Knight
Under Secretary
Marketing and Regulatory Programs

See comment 4.
See comment 5.

APPENDIX to USDA RESPONSE on
"Veterinarian Workforce: Actions Are Needed to Ensure
Sufficient Capacity for Protecting Public and Animal Health" (09-178)

**GENERAL COMMENTS ON GAO's
ANALYSIS OF FSIS OPERATIONS AND ACTIVITIES**

*Page 14, 1st sentence, last paragraph: It states that that "FSIS has never had a sufficient number of veterinarians..."*

**USDA Comment:** This is misleading. It would be more accurate to state that "Many FSIS veterinarian positions have gone unfilled due to a lack of candidates. In the past decade, FSIS has never been fully staffed with veterinarians..." On page 15, where it discusses vacancy rates, it would be more accurate and more in line with the information on page 14 to state that vacancy rates "varied by location and year, ranging from a very small percentage to as high as 35 percent of the total positions." Also, as GAO notes on page 15, FSIS has been able to reallocate veterinary resources sufficient to meet its statutory mandates for food safety and humane handling of livestock.

*Page 15, 2nd sentence, last paragraph: This sentence states that "Inhumane treatment of livestock contributed to the largest beef recall in US history, in February 2008."*

**USDA Comment:** As written, this sentence is factually incorrect. FSIS obtained evidence that the establishment did not consistently contact the FSIS public health veterinarian in situations in which cattle became non-ambulatory after passing ante-mortem inspection, which is not compliant with FSIS regulations. Such circumstances require that an FSIS public health veterinarian reassess the non-ambulatory cattle, which are either condemned and prohibited from the food supply, or tagged as suspect. It was this evidence that directly led to the voluntary recall by the Chino firm on February 17, 2008. The inhumane treatment was not the basis for the recall, but, rather, resulted in a suspension of operations which occurred on February 4, 2008. The inhumane treatment allegations were what led to the investigation into plant practices by USDA.

*Page 16, 2nd paragraph: This paragraph discusses instances of local veterinary shortages, and increased verification of humane handling.*

**USDA Comment:** Although FSIS has not been able to hire as many veterinarians in some locations as would be ideal, work is prioritized to ensure food safety tasks are performed. The full paragraph on p.16 should not give the impression that food safety is compromised by intermittent local veterinarian shortages. Veterinarians in FSIS are instructed to prioritize their time with food safety (which includes ante-mortem activities such as humane handling), then food defense activities being the highest priority. In the last few years, FSIS has placed supervisory consumer safety inspectors in many large slaughter plants. These employees directly report to the veterinarian, and provide significant relief to the supervisory activities of the veterinarian. This enables the veterinarians to focus their time on food safety related activities. From 2003 until 2008,

See comment 6.
See comment 7.

FSIS increased staffing for the number of SCSI's almost four fold, from 57 to 207. This paragraph also notes that "In the wake of this incident, FSIS required veterinarians to spend more tome verifying the humane treatment of animals". Although technically correct, as noted in FSIS Notice 17-08, this increased focus was for only a 60 day period between March 10 and May 6, 2008. During this brief period, it was important that humane handling activities took priority over other duties.

There is also much emphasis on the incidents at a plant in Chino, CA. This is attributed to having only one veterinarian assigned to the plant. It should be noted, however, that the incidents at this plant are not representative of FSIS regulatory control at comparable plants. FSIS is similarly staffed at comparable plants, but these incidents have not been replicated. In their recent audit report, OIG found no evidence of systematic humane handling problems. It is important to note, that the last time two veterinarians were assigned to the Chino facility was in the early 1990's. Simply because the plant slaughters cull cows is not a sufficiently justifiable reason to assign two veterinarians to a plant, especially following the ban on slaughter of downer cattle in late 2003 because the ante-mortem and post-mortem examination of downers was labor intensive.

*Page 16, last two sentences, 2nd paragraph: These last two sentences reference a recommendation made in a 2004 GAO report "...that FSIS periodically assess whether the level of resources dedicated to humane handling and slaughter activities is sufficient but the agency has yet to demonstrate that they have done so."*

**USDA Comment**. This same recommendation is repeated in the first paragraph on page 47 and again on page 48. It is our understanding that the recommendation from the 2004 GAO report, *Humane Methods of Slaughter Act: USDA Has Addressed Some Problems but Still Faces Enforcement Challenges*, has been closed. As stated in the response to the recommendation, FSIS already annually assesses its needs for the inspection and veterinary resources sufficient to meet its statutory mandates for food safety and the humane handling of livestock, as part of the budget formulation process. In addition, since the initial 2004 GAO report, FSIS has taken a number of actions in regard to ensuring the verification of compliance with the humane handling requirements. FSIS implemented the HATS database which is used by FSIS Public Health Veterinarians and other in-plant program personnel to report their time and data for specific humane handling activities. District Veterinary Medical Specialists (DVMS) routinely verify the accuracy of the data entered. For FY2008, FSIS inplant personnel spent approximately 120 FTE staff years, or 250,000 person-hours, verifying humane handling activities at the 800 livestock slaughter plants under Federal Inspection. Approximately 47% of this humane handling verification time was conducted by PHVs. Eighty-six humane handling related suspensions were effected at 65 of these livestock slaughter plants.

*Page 17: The first and second paragraphs on this page provide a comparison between the mean annual salary for FSIS veterinarians as compared to the mean salary for private practice veterinarians and discusses the steps FSIS has taken to address veterinary shortages.*

See comment 8.
See comment 9.

**USDA Comment:** We believe it should be noted that overtime work pushes the FSIS salaries closer to those in the private sector. We also believe, when discussing recruitment initiatives, the following should be included: "In April 2003 the FSIS and the Public Health Service (PHS) entered into a Memorandum of Agreement which significantly expanded the number of PHS Commissioned Corps Officers detailed to FSIS. The Commissioned Corps has a variety of occupations, including veterinarians, which help promote FSIS' public health mission. PHS Officers work as permanent staff members alongside their FSIS counterparts, and this has proven to be a valuable alternative method to fill vacant Veterinary Medical Officer positions."

*Page 18, last sentence, 1ˢᵗ paragraph: This sentence states that the "direct-hire authority" expired in 2007 and was not renewed.*

**USDA Comment:** On page 18, direct-hire information is outdated and incomplete. USDA submitted a request to resume using direct-hire authority, and the request was approved by OPM, on a limited basis, on November 25, 2008. FSIS will continue using this limited direct-hire authority for veterinarians at least through its December 31, 2009 expiration date. If recruitment difficulties continue, FSIS plans to request an extension of its direct-hire authority, without the limitations currently imposed. Currently, FSIS is limited to a total of 150 hires using this authority, and may only use it in locations where there are fewer than three eligible candidates. Given that it takes 5 to 6 months to obtain OPM approval, we will need to reinitiate our direct-hire request in July or August 2009 in hopes to have it approved prior to the December 31, 2009 expiration date. It would be more advantageous to the Agency if OPM would approve Government-wide direct hire authority for veterinarians without limitations and for a longer period of time than just one year.

*Page 26, Table 1: The table indicates that the veterinarian workforce falls short of Agency goals due to the unpleasant environment and grueling work.*

**USDA Comment:** The challenges faced by FSIS are not adequately highlighted. Recruitment difficulties result from more than the nature of the work and the work environment. In addition to what is already stated, it would be helpful to note that FSIS highlighted a wide variety of factors that have a negative impact on their recruitment efforts, including salary, lack of public health and food safety emphasis in Veterinary Colleges, and remote duty stations.

*Page 30, 1ˢᵗ paragraph: This paragraph discusses the change in the entry grade level for newly hired veterinarians and OPM's review of veterinarian classification initiated at USDA's request.*

**USDA Comment:** It should be noted that FSIS provided staff resources to expedite the development and implementation of the classification and qualification standards. The revised qualification standards were developed by an FSIS senior human resources specialist with input from all participating federal agencies. Additionally, during the development of the classification standard FSIS and APHIS veterinarians participated in focus groups, and both agencies reviewed the draft material in-depth at several stages. We recommend a minor change to the second sentence in the first paragraph: "This change paralleled the revised qualification standard for the veterinary occupation which raised the entry grade level for newly hired veterinarians from GS-9 to GS-11..." In addition, FSIS has been able to attract more veterinarians through the use of hiring flexibilities, such as superior qualifications, direct-hire authority and recruitment incentives."

*Page 30, 2^nd paragraph: This paragraph discusses NVMSA authority.*

**USDA Comment**: USDA funding under the NVMSA was rescinded 6/19/08. FSIS absorbed the student loan repayment obligations to the five individuals hired while under the NVMSA. Over a three-year period, it will cost the Agency a total of $150,000.

*Page 31, 5^th sentence, 2^nd paragraph: This sentence states that FEMA guidance directs agencies to identify three people who can carry out each responsibility and identify how the agency will continue to operate if leadership and essential staff are unavailable.*

**USDA Comment**: FSIS Human Pandemic Operations Plan (HPOP), Annex D shows that all program areas have identified at least 3 people who can carry out program responsibilities and ensure delivery of essential functions to the maximum extent possible with available personnel during an expected high rate of absenteeism during a pandemic. Section 2.1 of the HPOP details the essential functions of the program areas and alternate personnel (by job titles) who can take over the functions.

*Page 32, 3^rd sentence, 2^nd paragraph: The sentence states that FSIS' plan does not address the logistics on how FSIS will work with industry to ensure veterinarians and other employees are available in the event of a pandemic so that food production can continue.*

**USDA Comment**: FSIS is finalizing a Pandemic Resource Management Strategy developed in collaboration with the Food Sector Coordinating Council which outlines what the Agency and the Industry will do at the different stages of a pandemic to ensure food production is sustained to the maximum extent possible. FSIS actions include among other measures, the development of quick immersion training for veterinarians and other employees to ensure to the maximum extent possible that inspection services are provided that will allow the industry to produce food under continuous inspection. Priority allocation of resources to the slaughter inspection of certain species (poultry) may become necessary based on need identified through active communication with the industry. The Strategy will be added as an Annex to the HPOP.

*Page 33, 4^th sentence, 1^st paragraph: The sentence states that FSIS' plan does not mention how it would work with APHIS on activities related to surveillance of animal diseases.*

USDA Comment: In a pandemic, FSIS, as part of its essential inspection functions will continue to report foreign animal diseases, including BSE, that are of interest to APHIS as part of their surveillance program as per FSIS Directive 6000.1 (8/4/06) Responsibilities Related to Foreign Animal Diseases (FADS) and Reportable Conditions. Specific language will be added to the HPOP as part of its revision/update that is in progress

*Page 33, last sentence, 1ˢᵗ paragraph: The sentence states that FSIS' plan does not consider the impact of local quarantine on access to plants:*

USDA Comment: In a pandemic, FSIS does not intend to deploy inspection personnel from a non-pandemic area to a pandemic area. If quarantine is in effect however for a certain area, plant personnel will likewise be prevented from access to facilities therefore inspection services would not be needed. According to the Department guidance, FSIS inspection personnel may be granted special permission to enter local/State quarantine areas if deployment is deemed necessary, critical, and appropriate to provide inspection services.

The following are GAO's comments on the Department of Agriculture's letter dated January 16, 2009.

## GAO Comments

1. USDA commented that FSIS already regularly assesses the level of inspection resources it needs, as we recommended in 2004. However, as our report states, FSIS has yet to demonstrate that they have done so. We regularly follow up to request evidence that agencies have implemented our recommendations, and FSIS has not provided such evidence.

2. USDA reported the majority of its veterinarian workforce is located within two agencies, APHIS and FSIS, and each has the staff and expertise to conduct veterinarian workforce analyses for their respective agencies. Therefore, these two agencies will work together, with departmental consultation, as needed, to develop solutions to problems shared by both agencies. We continue to believe that a departmental assessment, not a consultation, is necessary, particularly in light of the competition between the two agencies. As we reported, APHIS is attracting veterinarians away from FSIS because the work at APHIS is more appealing, there are more opportunities for advancement, and the salaries are higher. Furthermore, ARS continues

to experience difficulties recruiting and retaining highly qualified veterinarians to carry out critical research of national importance, yet there is no mention of ARS in USDA's comments.

3. USDA commented that it has contingency plans and a decision tree for use of foot-and-mouth disease vaccine from the North American Foot-and-Mouth Disease Vaccine Bank. We acknowledge that USDA has these plans. In fact, we reviewed a draft plan titled, *Response to the Detection of Foot-and-Mouth Disease in the United States*, dated October 2007, that USDA officials told us was their new response plan that considered alternative response strategies, including "vaccinate to live." However, this plan does not detail how a policy of this nature would be implemented. USDA further commented that policy decisions as to who may administer the vaccine will be made based on the circumstances of the outbreak. While we recognize that each outbreak is unique, this should not preclude USDA from identifying a plausible scenario or scenarios and detailing how a vaccinate to live strategy would be carried out in order to enhance preparation, response, and recovery in a time of crises.

4. We modified our report to reflect that USDA would like to change their statement from FSIS has "never" had a sufficient number of veterinarians to "over the past decade." USDA also asserts that our report says that FSIS has been able to reallocate veterinary resources sufficient to meet its statutory mandates for food safety and humane handling of livestock. However, our report only presents this as the view of FSIS headquarters officials. We raise this point to illustrate that FSIS headquarters officials and veterinarians working in slaughter plants differ on the impact of this shortage.

5. We modified our report to reflect more clearly the relationship between the events at a Chino, California, plant and the February 2008 beef recall.

6. USDA commented that that our report emphasizes the incident at a plant in Chino, California. We raise the point because some veterinarians told us they did not have time to ensure the humane treatment of livestock, and this example illustrates inhumane treatment occurred despite the presence of FSIS inspectors. USDA further commented that we attribute this incident to having only one veterinarian. We do not state this in our report. We use this and other statements about resources to illustrate the need for FSIS to periodically assess whether the level of resources dedicated to humane

handling and slaughter activities is sufficient. They have yet to do so. In addition, USDA commented that the USDA Inspector General did not find systematic problems associated with oversight of humane handling at slaughter facilities that process cull cows. However, the Inspector General did conclude that there is inherent vulnerability at the other plants in the scope of its audit, and that inhumane handling could occur and not be detected by FSIS inspectors due to lack of continuous surveillance.

7.  USDA commented that GAO has closed the 2004 recommendation that FSIS periodically assess whether the level of resources dedicated to humane handling and slaughter activities is sufficient. We recognize that FSIS has taken actions in response to a number of recommendations made in the 2004 report and have documented implementation of these recommendations. However, with regard to periodic assessment, we closed this recommendation because enough time had passed that we considered it unlikely to be implemented. As our report states, FSIS has yet to demonstrate that it has been implemented. Based on our current work, we continue to believe that periodic assessment is needed, and we make a recommendation to that effect.

8.  We modified our report to include the recent approval of USDA's direct-hire authority and noted that USDA has raised some concerns.

9.  We modified our report to include the concern about veterinary schools and enhanced the chart to include the concern for salary.

In: Veterinarian Workforce Role in Defense...       ISBN: 978-1-60741-656-2
Editor: Justin C. Bennett                                © 2010 Nova Science Publishers, Inc.

*Chapter 12*

# APPENDIX IV: COMMENTS FROM THE DEPARTMENT OF DEFENSE

## *United States Government Accountability Office*

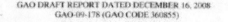

GAO DRAFT REPORT DATED DECEMBER 16, 2008
GAO-09-178 (GAO CODE 360855)

"VETERINARIAN WORKFORCE: ACTIONS ARE NEEDED TO
ENSURE SUFFICIENT CAPACITY FOR PROTECTING PUBLIC AND
ANIMAL HEALTH"

DEPARTMENT OF DEFENSE COMMENTS
TO THE GAO RECOMMENDATION

RECOMMENDATION: In report recommendation number 5 the GAO recommends that the
Secretary of Defense ensure that the component agencies that employ veterinarians complete
pandemic plans that contain the necessary elements put forth in the Department of Homeland
Security's continuity of operations pandemic guidance, including periodically testing, training,
and exercising plans.

DOD RESPONSE: Concur. As reflected in the draft report, DoD is currently working with
component agencies that employ veterinarians to complete pandemic plans that contain the
necessary elements of the Department of Homeland Security's continuity of operations pandemic
guidance (including periodically testing, training, and exercising plans). Efforts are underway to
finalize the Army Pandemic Influenza (PI) Plan. The Emergency Preparedness and Response
Branch, Headquarters, US Army MEDCOM, plans to hold a 2nd Quarter, FY 2009
conference/teleconference for all concerned parties to adjust the current Army plan to meet the
NORTHCOM-directed PI response phases. The implementation date of the final PI plan will be
determined based on current mission priorities.

In: Veterinarian Workforce Role in Defense...       ISBN: 978-1-60741-656-2
Editor: Justin C. Bennett                           © 2010 Nova Science Publishers, Inc.

**Chapter 13**

# APPENDIX V: COMMENTS FROM THE DEPARTMENT OF HEALTH AND HUMAN SERVICES

## *United States Government Accountability Office*

Note: GAO comments supplementing those in the report text appear at the end of this appendix.

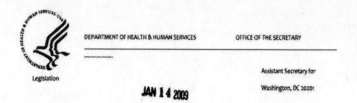

DEPARTMENT OF HEALTH & HUMAN SERVICES          OFFICE OF THE SECRETARY

Legislation

JAN 1 4 2009

Assistant Secretary for

Washington, DC 20201

Lisa Shames
Director, Natural Resources and Environment
U.S. Government Accountability Office
441 G Street N.W.
Washington, DC 20548

Dear Ms. Shames:

Enclosed are comments on the U.S. Government Accountability Office's (GAO) report entitled: "Veterinarian Workforce: Actions Are Needed to Ensure Sufficient Capacity for Protecting Public and Animal Health" (GAO-09-178).

The Department appreciates the opportunity to review this report before its publication.

Sincerely,

Craig Burton
Acting Assistant Secretary for Legislation

See comment 1.
See comment 2.

**COMMENTS OF THE DEPARTMENT OF HEALTH AND HUMAN SERVICES (HHS) ON THE GOVERNMENT ACCOUNTABILITY OFFICE'S (GAO) DRAFT REPORT ENTITLED: VETERINARIAN WORKFORCE ACTIONS ARE NEEDED TO ENSURE SUFFICIENT CAPACITY FOR PROTECTING PUBLIC AND ANIMAL HEALTH (GAO-09-178)**

The Department of Health and Human Services (HHS) appreciates the opportunity to review and comment on the General Accountability Office's (GAO) Draft Report entitled, "Veterinarian Workforce Actions Are Needed to Ensure Sufficient Capacity for Protecting Public and Animal Health (GAO-09-178)." We recognize that veterinarians are essential to protecting the health of the American people.

**GENERAL COMMENTS:**

While the veterinary series is not currently identified as a Department level Mission Critical Occupation (MCO) due largely to veterinarians representing less than one (1) percent of the HHS workforce, the Department plans to review its MCOs in the coming year according to a more risk based set of criteria.

In an agency as decentralized and diverse as HHS, HHS has taken an operating-division-centric approach to workforce planning. All operating and staff division heads are required to have workforce plans in place for their organizations by September 2009. The Department also plans to strengthen its oversight of the operating divisions to ensure that they are implementing their workforce plans, focusing on those occupations critical to the success of their missions.

The Department however, disagrees with GAO's premise that controlling zoonotic diseases is solely dependent on the capacity of the veterinarian workforce. CDC's zoonotic outbreak response strategy is robust and is not limited to veterinarians (DVM/VMD), but also involves persons with other professional degrees (MPH, PhD, MD). Likewise, veterinarians as well as these professionals from other disciplines serve in various roles as epidemiologists, health communicators, laboratorians, animal care technicians, and public health advisors. In the Technical Comments, we provide clarification that insufficient veterinarian capacity was not a workforce challenge in the responses to the monkeypox and West Nile virus outbreaks. That being said, veterinarians are a valuable resource at CDC and conducting regular workforce assessments, as recommended in the GAO report, will ensure that we maintain a sufficient capacity for outbreak responses.

The same example holds true in the Office of the Assistant Secretary for Preparedness and Response (ASPR). ASPR ensures a coordinated approach to public health emergencies and medical disaster preparedness and response capability by leading and coordinating the relevant activities of the HHS Operating Divisions on behalf of, and subject to the authority of, the Secretary.

ASPR also leads the Department for *Emergency Support Function (ESF) #8 – Public Health and Medical Services* (ESF #8), in the event of a public health emergency or medical disaster, ASPR coordinates the provision of federal public health and medical assistance (via HHS assets and ESF#8 partner/supporting agencies, departments,

See comment 3.
See comment 4.

organizations) to fulfill the requirements identified by the affected state and local authorities in several areas, including veterinary and/or animal health issues.

Disaster and emergency response programs are developed by teams of subject matter experts with a variety of skills and technical backgrounds (not only veterinarians) including microbiologists, epidemiologists, physicians, etc whose training and expertise may include areas overlapping with those of veterinarians. Veterinarians may bring additional expertise and should be sought for enhancing the overall perspective and depth of response planning.

The mission of ASPR's Emergency System for Advance Registration of Volunteer Health Professionals (ESAR-VHP) program is to establish and maintain a national network of state-based systems for advance registration of health professionals for the purpose of verifying the credentials, licenses, accreditations, and hospital privileges of such professionals, when, during public health emergencies, the professionals volunteer to provide health services. This national network of systems allows for the management of volunteer health professionals at all tiers of response (local, state, regional, and federal). All state ESAR-VHP systems are required to have the ability to register and collect the credentials and qualifications of veterinarians.

Successful recruitment of veterinarians at NIH poses an additional hurdle that the report did not identify - board specialization in laboratory animal medicine. Achieving specialty in laboratory animal medicine is very difficult (~40% pass rate). Also, very few veterinarians are interested in accruing additional debt immediately upon graduation from veterinary school in order to enter a residency program.

The Department does not agree with the statement cited on page 21, referencing the 2007 Science Board report, characterizing the FDA's Center for Veterinary Medicine (CVM) as being "in a state of crisis." Given the broad nature of the 2007 Science Board report (i.e., the report addressed, among other things, CVM's scientific workforce in general), the suggestion that these conclusions necessarily applied to CVM's veterinary workforce in particular is a misstatement. Furthermore, CVM has made great strides in the past few years in assessing its workforce needs and has implemented effective strategies for recruiting and retaining the finest workforce possible. The conclusions of the report are out of date in that they do not take into account the many workforce-related activities undertaken by CVM since 2007.

As a participant in the comprehensive Agency Food Protection Plan and Import Strategy initiatives for protecting the nation's food supply, CVM has outlined its needs to close the resource gap in order to function at full potential. In addition, as part of the Animal Drug User Fee Act (ADUFA) and the Animal Generic Drug User Fee Act (AGDUFA) analysis, CVM outlined the resources needed to meet statutory review timeframes and meet industry and public expectations. Finally, this past year CVM completed a gap

**COMMENTS OF THE DEPARTMENT OF HEALTH AND HUMAN SERVICES (HHS) ON THE GOVERNMENT ACCOUNTABILITY OFFICE'S (GAO) DRAFT REPORT ENTITLED: VETERINARIAN WORKFORCE ACTIONS ARE NEEDED TO ENSURE SUFFICIENT CAPACITY FOR PROTECTING PUBLIC AND ANIMAL HEALTH (GAO-09-178)**

analysis for all of its programs to measure the "gap" between current and optimal performance and the resources required to close the gap. This ensures CVM resources are appropriately aligned with current and future needs.

Through an integrated and coordinated process, CVM has built alliances and partnerships with private and governmental groups and has developed a recruitment process, which includes attending job fairs at universities and trade shows. These activities have enabled CVM to exceed the Agency's Hiring Surge goals.

With the enactment of AGDUFA, CVM is hiring staff to enhance the performance of the generic new animal drug review process. This will reduce the time required for safe and effective generic animal drugs to reach the marketplace, which provides consumers a lower cost alternative to pioneer drugs. Under AGDUFA, the new hires help FDA to meet specified performance goals over five (5) years for review of certain submissions.

Over a five (5) year period (FY2004 - FY2008) CVM hired 56 Full Time Equivalent Employees, which helped CVM meet or exceed all of its ADUFA performance goals for applications and submissions each year. In FY2008, for the first time in over a decade, CVM met and surpassed all its statutory timeframes.

Moreover, the Department does not agree with the statement in reference to (Page 21) the report that "veterinarians enter FDA employment lacking necessary skills and experience to examine the wide variety of veterinary products that require FDA approval and that FDA needs to better train its veterinarians to review the many diverse products under its jurisdiction."

CVM has been very successful in attracting, hiring, and retaining highly qualified veterinarians. Veterinarians hired by CVM qualify under a variety of "occupational series" and many of them come to CVM with significant scientific and clinical experience as well as advanced educational backgrounds in addition to the Doctor of Veterinary Medicine degree (e.g., Ph.D., M.P.H., M.B.A., J.D.).

CVM's Succession Plan offers a wide variety of programs for new and current employees to support them in their efforts to reach their maximum potential by strengthening and increasing their professional competencies. The CVM Succession Plan is embedded into a Competency Model, a tool that helps CVM determine what skills are required in particular job roles/functions to meet the present requirements of the organization, and most importantly, the needs of the future.

Furthermore, all CVM employees have access to a robust training program made available through CVM's Staff College. The CVM Staff College directs the development and implementation of the competency-based management and leadership development programs. The extensive scientific and regulatory curricula that include veterinary drug

See comment 5.

COMMENTS OF THE DEPARTMENT OF HEALTH AND HUMAN SERVICES
(HHS) ON THE GOVERNMENT ACCOUNTABILITY OFFICE'S (GAO) DRAFT
REPORT ENTITLED: VETERINARIAN WORKFORCE ACTIONS ARE
NEEDED TO ENSURE SUFFICIENT CAPACITY FOR PROTECTING PUBLIC
AND ANIMAL HEALTH (GAO-09-178)

law bring CVM veterinarians and scientists up to speed on applying the appropriate
regulatory law to the drug review process of veterinary products. The Staff College
collaborates with outside experts from industry and the academia such as the University of
Maryland, Baltimore, who keep CVM scientists and veterinary reviewers informed on
emerging science and technology. The Staff College continues to expand its training
initiatives as seen with its collaboration with other FDA Centers and federal agencies requiring
similar skill sets and sharing similar issues. The CVM Staff College also makes every effort
to obtain accreditation for continuing education credits from the Maryland State Board
for Veterinary Medicine for all scientific and emerging technology seminars offered.

The Department would like to clarify the statements in reference to (Page 21) of the
report indicating that "Although FDA officials said the veterinary workforce is sufficient,
CVM officials recently told us that the Center hired 26 veterinarians in 2008 to fill
vacancies" (17% increase in FDA's overall veterinarian workforce) "and it plans to hire
more."

In responding to survey questions provided as part of the GAO study that focused
primarily on the adequacy of the veterinary workforce for responding to zoonotic disease
outbreaks, CVM did indicate that it had a sufficient number of veterinarians to respond to
such occurrences. As described in the survey question response, FDA's veterinary
expertise resides primarily at FDA headquarters with the greatest concentration within
CVM. If an issue regarding a zoonotic disease arises, the veterinary resources in the
Agency are tapped as needed to address the issue. This approach has proven to be an
effective means for utilizing this expertise when the need arises. Furthermore, the
primary role of FDA veterinarians in responding to zoonotic disease outbreaks is to
provide technical/scientific advice and to coordinate FDA's activities with those of other
federal, state, and local agencies. In light of their role as coordinators and consultants in
such situations, we believe FDA has a sufficient number of veterinarians on staff that
could be temporarily reassigned as needed to respond to such an event.

Subsequent to responding to the aforementioned survey question, CVM proceeded with
its ongoing efforts to assess its resource needs to address changes in its current workforce
(e.g., backfill vacancies/attrition) and to address new workforce demands associated with
newly acquired responsibilities. In particular, during this timeframe CVM took on a
number of new obligations including those associated with the agency's Food Protection
Plan, the FDA Amendments Act, and the Animal Generic Drug User Fee Act. Therefore,
the significant increase observed in CVM's veterinary workforce was primarily in
response to these new obligations. CVM plans to continue its workforce assessment and
gap analysis to determine staffing that may be required to support workload related to
other emerging issues and technologies (e.g., nanotechnology, biotechnology).

GAO made nine (9) *Recommendations for Executive Action* to improve the ability of the
federal veterinarian workforce to carry out routine activities, prepare for a catastrophic

**COMMENTS OF THE DEPARTMENT OF HEALTH AND HUMAN SERVICES (HHS) ON THE GOVERNMENT ACCOUNTABILITY OFFICE'S (GAO) DRAFT REPORT ENTITLED:VETERINARIAN WORKFORCE ACTIONS ARE NEEDED TO ENSURE SUFFICIENT CAPACITY FOR PROTECTING PUBLIC AND ANIMAL HEALTH (GAO-09-178)**

event, and respond to zoonotic disease outbreaks. We offer general comment(s) regarding four (4) GAO recommendations, which specifically address the Department (pages 48 and 49 of the draft report).

Third, Eighth and Ninth GAO recommendation – that the Secretary of HHS direct the department's component agencies that employ veterinarians to conduct regular workforce assessments, and that the Secretary then conduct a department-wide assessment of HHS's veterinarian workforce to identify current and future workforce needs (including training and employee development) and solutions to problems shared by its agencies. When HHS completes its assessment, it should forward the results to the Director of OPM.

In a department as decentralized and diverse as HHS, HHS has taken an operating division centric approach to workforce planning. All operating and staff division heads are required to have workforce plans in place for their organizations by September 2009. Once the plans are in completed, the HHS Office of Human Resources will look across the plans to identify opportunities for collaboration with regard to strategic recruitment, development and retention. The department also plans to strengthen its oversight of the operating divisions to ensure that they are implementing their workforce plans, focusing on those occupations critical to the success of their missions.

Fifth GAO recommendation – The Secretaries of Agriculture, Defense, and Health and Human Services ensure that their component agencies that employ veterinarians complete pandemic plans that contain the necessary elements put forth in DHS's continuity of operations pandemic guidance, including periodically testing, training, and exercising plans.

HHS concurs with this recommendation. Work currently underway at the HHS Food and Drug Administration (FDA) provides an illustration of how HHS is addressing this recommendation through one of its component agencies.

As part of FDA's follow-up and after actions to the October 2008 *FDA Pandemic Influenza Functional Exercise,* the agency will be updating its *FDA Pandemic Influenza Emergency Response Plan.* The update will include addressing the necessary elements put forth in DHS's continuity of operations pandemic guidance. The specific elements that will be addressed include:

- identifying what essential functions performed by veterinarians must be performed on-site;
- delegation of authority to three individuals capable of carrying out each essential function performed by veterinarians;
- contact information for individuals who could assume authority should essential veterinarian staff and leadership become unavailable; and

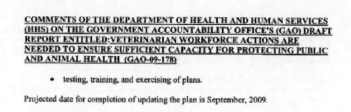

**COMMENTS OF THE DEPARTMENT OF HEALTH AND HUMAN SERVICES (HHS) ON THE GOVERNMENT ACCOUNTABILITY OFFICE'S (GAO) DRAFT REPORT ENTITLED:VETERINARIAN WORKFORCE ACTIONS ARE NEEDED TO ENSURE SUFFICIENT CAPACITY FOR PROTECTING PUBLIC AND ANIMAL HEALTH (GAO-09-178)**

- testing, training, and exercising of plans.

Projected date for completion of updating the plan is September, 2009.

As a side note, the FDA Pandemic Influenza Operational Annex to the *HHS Pandemic Influenza Operational Plan* provides extensive guidance to agency officials on ways to mitigate the impact of high absenteeism and to ensure continued operations and coverage for essential functions. Examples from the Annex include:

- Re-employment of annuitants;
- SES Limited Emergency Appointments; and
- One-year temporary emergency need appointments.

The following are GAO's comments on the Department of Health and Human Services' letter dated January 14, 2009.

## GAO Comments

1. HHS commented that a premise of our report is that the control of zoonotic diseases is solely dependent on the capacity of the veterinarian workforce. Our report does not state this. The scope of this report, as described in the introduction, was to review the sufficiency of the federal veterinarian workforce.
2. Our report does not identify the Centers for Disease Control and Prevention (CDC) as having too few veterinarians to control the 2003 West Nile virus outbreak while also adequately carrying out other

routine activities. However, CDC officials we interviewed who were involved with the 2003 monkeypox outbreak in Wisconsin told us there were too few veterinarians during this outbreak.

3.  We modified our report to reflect the new information about the difficulty the National Institutes of Health has recruiting veterinarians.

4.  Our report states conclusions from the FDA Advisory Committee report: that FDA "cannot fulfill its mission" because its scientific workforce has remained static while its workload has increased, and that FDA's Center for Veterinary Medicine (CVM) is "in a state of crisis." We discussed with an author of the Advisory Committee report how that report's findings specifically related to veterinarians. Consequently, our report also states that an author of the FDA Advisory Committee report told us that veterinarians enter FDA employment lacking necessary skills and experience to examine the wide variety of veterinary products that require FDA approval and that FDA needs to better train its veterinarians to review the many diverse products under its jurisdiction. HHS further stated that CVM has made great strides in the past few years in assessing its workforce needs and that the conclusions of the Advisory Committee report are out of date. Our report identifies several of the efforts CVM has recently undertaken, such as hiring additional veterinarians and beginning efforts to analyze the gap between current resources and needs. It also notes that, according to FDA officials, the agency is undertaking significant reforms to address fundamental concerns in the 2007 report. However, as our report states, FDA did not tell us how these efforts address the identified veterinarian skill gap specifically.

5.  We modified our report to add a statement that the increase observed in CVM's veterinarian workforce was primarily in response to new obligations.

In: Veterinarian Workforce Role in Defense...          ISBN: 978-1-60741-656-2
Editor: Justin C. Bennett                    © 2010 Nova Science Publishers, Inc.

*Chapter 14*

# APPENDIX VI: COMMENTS FROM THE OFFICE OF PERSONNEL MANAGEMENT

## *United States Government Accountability Office*

Note: GAO comments supplementing those in the report text appear at the end of this appendix.

See comment 1. See comment 2.

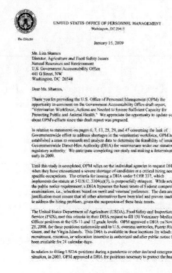

Ms. Lisa Shames

safety of the U.S. food supply. This DHA allows the USDA to fill temporary and term positions in a variety of occupational categories, including Veterinary Medical Officers at the GS-9 through 13 grade levels. This DHA is limited to non-permanent positions because these excess employees would no longer be needed upon recovery from the pandemic or termination of the emergency.

We also note that under 5 CFR 213.3102(i)(3), OPM may allow agencies to temporarily appoint individuals in the excepted service during a pandemic or emergency situation. OPM permitted agencies to use this authority to immediately staff emergency positions in the aftermaths of September 11, 2001, and Hurricanes Katrina and Rita.

Technical comments to the draft report are enclosed. Unless otherwise noted, the suggested revisions are meant to provide technical accuracy and conform to terminology applicable to the Federal service.

Please contact Mr. David Cushing on (202) 606-4660 should your office require additional information.

Again, my thanks to your office for providing this opportunity to update and clarify information in the draft report.

Sincerely,

Michael W. Hagar
Acting Director

Enclosure

The following are GAO's comments on the Office of Personnel Management's letter dated January 15, 2009.

## GAO Comments

1. We modified our report to reflect OPM's establishment of a team to determine the feasibility of issuing a governmentwide direct-hire authority for veterinarians.
2. We modified our report to include OPM's recent approval of USDA's direct-hire authority request.

In: Veterinarian Workforce Role in Defense...      ISBN: 978-1-60741-656-2
Editor: Justin C. Bennett                           © 2010 Nova Science Publishers, Inc.

*Chapter 15*

# APPENDIX VII: COMMENTS FROM THE DEPARTMENT OF HOMELAND SECURITY

## *United States Government Accountability Office*

Note: GAO comments supplementing those in the report text appear at the end of this appendix.

U.S. Department of Homeland Security
Washington, DC 20528

**Homeland Security**

January 14, 2009

Ms. Lisa Shames
Director, Natural Resources and Environment
U.S. Government Accountability Office
441 G Street, NW
Washington, DC 20548

Dear Ms. Shames:

RE: Draft Report GAO-09-178, *Veterinarian Workforce: Actions Are Needed to Ensure Sufficient Capacity for Protecting Public and Animal Health.*

Thank you for the opportunity to review and comment on the Government Accountability Office's (GAO's) Draft Report GAO-09-178 entitled *Veterinarian Workforce: Actions Are Needed to Ensure Sufficient Capacity for Protecting Public and Animal Health.* We concur with the recommendation that applies to the Department of Homeland Security. We have included comments and additional recommendations for your consideration.

**General Comments:**

GAO states that they are making several recommendations to improve the federal government's ability to meet its routine veterinary responsibilities.

The report states: "The federal government has undertaken efforts to identify the veterinarian workforce needed during two catastrophic events—a pandemic and multiple intentional introductions of foot-and-mouth disease. However, these efforts are limited in their usefulness because they are either incomplete, based on an infeasible planning assumption, or lacking adequate data." DHS concurs in part, and proposes the following additional language:

> "We recommend that the federal government enhance efforts to identify the veterinary workforce. This may be achieved through an OPM pursuit of a multi-department assessment of veterinary manpower requirements to include an all-hazards approach with regards to requirements for prevention, preparation, response, and recovery."

In section, *Pandemic;* the report states, " Four of the five agencies we reviewed—APHIS, FSIS, ARS, and FDA — have developed plans that identify how they will continue essential functions, including those that veterinarians perform, during a pandemic that

www.dhs.gov

See comment 1.
See comment 2.

severely reduces the workforce. However, each plan lacks elements that DHS has deemed necessary." DHS concurs in part, and proposes the following additional language:

> "We recommend that agencies develop plans that identify how they will continue essential functions during additional catastrophic events, taking into consideration the potential for greater than the estimated 40 percent absenteeism during a pandemic. We also recommend, that once an overall government-wide veterinary manpower needs determination is made, that the government directs its efforts to developing effective recruitment and retention programs."

Under the section, *Foot-and-mouth disease outbreak* the report refers to an infeasible planning assumption that the United States would slaughter all potentially exposed animals as it has during smaller outbreaks of foreign animal diseases, and that the resultant workforce estimates (required to implement the infeasible planning assumption) are not relevant. DHS does not concur that the workforce estimates are not relevant; the current policy requires slaughter of all potentially exposed animals and therefore the projected manpower requirement is relevant.

DHS agrees that this approach may be infeasible for a large foot-and-mouth outbreak. Procedures that accurately describe a catastrophic foot-and-mouth disease incident and appropriate response would be beneficial. DHS proposes that the following language be deleted:

> "However, DHS and USDA officials consider this approach infeasible for such a large outbreak and told us that although the planning effort is a valuable exercise for understanding the enormity of the resources needed to respond to such an event, any workforce estimates produced from this effort are not relevant."

DHS proposes that the following language is inserted:

> "Even though DHS and USDA officials consider this approach infeasible for a catastrophic foot-and-mouth disease incident, the planning effort is necessary because the slaughter of all potentially exposed animals remains the currently accepted response to a foot-and-mouth disease outbreak."

In the chart on Homeland Security, column on Examples of Concerns, DHS proposes that the following language be deleted:

> "Pool of candidates with the skills necessary to help plan for the defense of the nation's food supply is small; office lacks the resources to offer salaries sufficient to attract such veterinarians."

DHS proposes that the following language is inserted:

"Veterinary expertise contributes to agriculture, animal health and human health. The agency has too few veterinarians to effectively develop the capabilities to respond to catastrophic food, agriculture, and veterinary events."

Following that chart, the report states that retirement within the next 3 years would be approximately 27 percent which would exacerbate the shortage of veterinarians in the federal agencies. DHS concurs and proposes the following additional language:

"Based on these figures, we recommend that the government direct its efforts to develop effective recruitment and retention programs."

DHS Office of Health Affairs (OHA) submits the following background information. OHA stood up on March 31, 2007. The OHA mission includes developing a robust biological threat awareness capacity and information sharing with food and agriculture communities, enhancing local response capabilities for agro-defense and collaborating with other federal agencies to prevent introduction of foreign animal and plant pathogens into this country. In order to accomplish this mission, OHA, filled senior level veterinary positions first with the intention of filling entry level positions later. When this is accomplished, OHA average salaries will be within range of other agency veterinary positions in the Washington D.C. metropolitan area.

Referring to the paragraph after Figure 3 and Note: the report states: "Some agencies, such as those within HHS and the Department of Veterans Affairs, can augment base salaries for veterinarians using special statutory authorities." DHS concurs and proposes the following additional language:

"OPM should consistently apply incentive programs across all agencies for recruitment and retention of veterinarians."

Technical comments have been provided under separate cover.

Sincerely,

Jerald E. Levine
Director
Departmental GAO/OIG Liaison

The following are GAO's comments on the Department of Homeland Security's letter dated January 14, 2009.

## GAO Comments

1. DHS stated that current policy requires slaughter of all potentially exposed animals and, therefore, the projected manpower requirement is relevant. We agree that this estimate is relevant to this method. As our report notes, the United States has used this "stamping out" method in the past for eradicating smaller outbreaks of foreign animal diseases. However, DHS and USDA officials told us, and DHS reiterates in its comments, that stamping out is infeasible for a large-scale outbreak of foot-and-mouth disease. Therefore, we do not agree that this estimate is relevant to a catastrophic outbreak, which was the scope of this section of our report. Indeed, as we note, DHS and USDA officials we interviewed during the course of our review told us that the estimate was not relevant.

2. We modified our report to clarify the Office of Health Affairs' concerns about the sufficiency of its veterinarian workforce.

In: Veterinarian Workforce Role in Defense...          ISBN: 978-1-60741-656-2
Editor: Justin C. Bennett                          © 2010 Nova Science Publishers, Inc.

Chapter 16

# APPENDIX VIII: COMMENTS FROM THE DEPARTMENT OF THE INTERIOR

## United States Government Accountability Office

Comments from the Department of the Interior on the U.S. Government Accountability Office (GAO) draft report entitled, *"VETERINARIAN WORKFORCE Actions Are Needed to Ensure Sufficient Capacity for Protecting Public and Animal Health"*
Report Number GAO-09-178

We agree with the recommendations and wish to emphasize the importance of including wildlife disease expertise and resources into the strategy for protecting human and animal health.

DOI's veterinarians and disease experts bring to bear a diverse array of scientific expertise that compliment and enhance the work of other agencies. DOI leadership in wildlife health activities helps assure a truly integrated approach to protecting the health of human and wild and domestic animals. A comprehensive approach that includes wildlife is critical for facilitating early detection and timely intervention of emerging infectious diseases, which can impact humans.

Emerging zoonotic diseases such as the West Nile Virus and Ebola appeared first in wildlife, gaining a foothold in wildlife populations before spilling over into humans. Interior wildlife disease surveillance and infrastructure proactively address wildlife disease. The Department of Homeland Security has expressed concern that wildlife could be used by terrorists as potential "delivery systems" for the introduction of pathogens into human and domestic animal populations. Current DOI wildlife disease activities and research such as DOI's Avian Influenza surveillance in migratory wild birds could also potentially detect intentionally introduced pathogens and/or help discern naturally occurring disease events from intentional introductions.

A related topic that is not addressed in the GAO report but that we feel is key to protecting human, animal, and ecosystem health as well as economic interests within the U.S. borders is the detection and prevention of non-native invasive infectious agents from entering U.S. borders via imported wildlife. The recent Monkey Pox outbreak illustrates how quickly an infectious disease from imported animals can be disseminated around the country. Interior's FWS port inspection program is key to detecting and containing pathogens before an imported animal enters the country providing the best opportunity for preventing disease outbreaks.

During the importation process a single sick animal has the potential to infect a large number of animals in the same shipment. In addition, the mixing of animals during the importation process also provides an ideal environment for "new" diseases to develop. Diseases such as Ebola, HIV/AIDS and Mad Cow disease all developed as a result of pathogen moving from its normal host species into a new species.

To adequately address these areas Interior needs to evaluate workforce needs that could support: (1) Research - including identifying and developing alternative methods such as risk assessments for screening animals when diagnostic tests are not available or not feasible, (2) testing and/or necropsying suspect animals when appropriate, and (3) providing the U.S. Ports of Entry and Border Offices additional personnel and training to detect and sample for disease in wildlife species.

At the Federal level we recommend that a part of the workforce planning be focused on capacity building including specialized, multidisciplinary training for wildlife veterinarians including clinical diseases of wildlife, ecology, wildlife epidemiology, and environmental health. We also recommend that predictive disease models, such as those developed for Foot and Mouth disease and plague, include wildlife species when appropriate. As the GAO report correctly points out, models that address only captive animals will be inadequate. Disease prevention and control methods developed for use in captive/controlled agriculture will likely be ineffective and not feasible if free ranging wildlife are involved in the outbreak. For that reason it is critical to have wildlife disease specialists including ecologists, and epidemiologists involved in the development of the disease models and the response plans.

# INDEX